TYPE 1
DIABETES
AND HOW TO LIVE WITH IT

by Paul Coker

ISBN: 978-1910202067

First published 2014

Typeset for The Write Family Ltd by Kir Lysenka.

Printed in Great Britain for The Book Publishing Academy by Bell & Bain Ltd, 303 Burnfield Road, Thornliebank, Glasgow G46 7UQ.

CONTENTS

DISCLAIMER

This book is not intended as a substitute for the medical advice of physicians. The reader should regularly consult a physician in matters relating to his/her health, and particularly with respect to any symptoms that may require diagnosis or medical attention. No warranties are made, expressed, or implied, with regard to the contents of this book or is applicability to specific individuals. The authors and publishers shall not be liable for direct, indirect, special, incidental or consequential damages arising out of the use of or inability to use the contents of this book. Never use this book on your own! Any suggestion in this book for improving diabetes management should only be followed under the guidance of your healthcare team. Never under estimate the importance of good professional advice and support. No book can ever help you as much as your health care professionals; together you make a fantastic team.

CHAPTER ONE

INTRODUCTION

Type 1 diabetes has been part of my life every day since I was diagnosed in the summer of 1977 when I was just five years old. Every day since my life has revolved around the medical aspects of the disease: numbers; calculating insulin doses; analysing food for its carbohydrate content, fat content, fibre content; measuring the volume of glucose in my urine, because in the early days blood glucose testing was not available in the home setting; and then later measuring my blood glucose levels. Let's not forget about the 50,000 injections that have kept me alive and the 60,000 hours (and counting) that I have been connected to an insulin pump. During all of this time the outside world has viewed type 1 diabetes as being very simple to manage. "If you just take your insulin injections, you will be fine".

Even if you have only been living with diabetes for a few hours you probably know that insulin injections will keep you alive, but living with type 1 diabetes means that you no longer have the innate ability to maintain normal blood glucose levels. If your blood glucose levels are running too high you may feel like you have the flu and, if they are not managed, you will develop a life-threatening condition called Diabetic Ketoacidosis. However, if your blood glucose levels are too low, you will experience low blood glucose levels, also known as hypoglycaemia. This condition leads to impairment of cognitive function and makes it seem like you are drunk – left untreated this situation is also fatal. As a person with diabetes you suddenly become aware that the quest for stable blood glucose levels is almost like the quest for the holy grail.

In my own particular case a doctor failed to diagnose my diabetes at the age of five, even though I had presented with every classic symptom, meaning my body was shutting down and I was dying. When I was seven years old I was admitted to hospital for minor elective surgery, whilst the surgery went well, the lack of understanding about diabetes threatened my life once more; in fact, my life was saved by the intervention of my mother, and I was discharged from hospital whilst still in Diabetic Ketoacidosis because they could not cope with my diabetes. Whilst I was recovering from this surgery at home I realised that I had been lucky, but if I was going to survive with diabetes, I would need to be an expert in my own condition. At the tender age of seven I started to read everything that I could find about diabetes as though my life depended upon it, remember we did not have the Internet back then, I would go to the library and get medical reference books and encyclopaedias to expand my knowledge. My passion for life and learning about diabetes has been with me since that day. I remain grateful to the incompetence of those doctors early in my life because they inspired me to gain more knowledge about diabetes.

Many people with diabetes, who know of my condition and have seen the way in which I live my life, have asked me questions on how I manage diabetes with my busy schedule because they want to know how to manage their own diabetes. It is because of these questions that I am writing this book – I love to talk to people about diabetes and I love to help. I can do this on a one-to-one basis, in small groups, in person or over the Internet, but in writing this book, I can reach out and educate, support, and empower more people who are living with type 1 diabetes. This book is written for everyone whose life is impacted by this metabolic disease, whether it's for yourself or for your son, daughter, husband, wife, partner, or friend who has the condition. I have included a section on how friends and family can offer support. There is nothing worse than well-meaning relatives and friends policing the way I manage my diabetes, I don't need their judgements, but I do need their love and support. I share some of my philosophies on living with diabetes and on how to manage the physical aspects. I also share my insight on how I manage the mental impact of living with a lifelong debilitating, yet invisible condition.

Dr Joslin was the first American doctor to specialise in diabetes care in 1908, 14 years before insulin was isolated, and yet he had an incredible insight and is famously quoted as saying **"the patient who knows the most about diabetes lives the longest"**. Unfortunately the availability of formal education for people with diabetes about diabetes is severely lacking, and healthcare agencies all over the world appear to be struggling to deliver the necessary education to allow people with type 1 diabetes to develop the strategies they need to live full, active and independent lives. My own philosophy is an extension of this: **Education leads to Empowerment**. My knowledge of diabetes and how to live with it allows me to be a father and husband, have a successful full-time career, invest time in helping the Juvenile Diabetes Research Foundation (JDRF) to raise funds for the research into a cure for diabetes, represent INPUT Diabetes (a charity which advocates for people with diabetes) at the Welsh Assembly, run half marathons, take part in some incredible personal challenges, and give presentations about living with diabetes, provide support and coaching to people with diabetes and, of course, write books about type 1 diabetes.

I am honoured that you have chosen to read my book and I respect you as a person who wants to live an extraordinary life, knowing that diabetes will not prevent you and yours from achieving whatever goals you decide to set for yourself. The best athletes and sports people have professionals to help them improve their game. It gives them a short cut to success. It is my view that all of us need a coach to learn from as we are not born with an in-depth knowledge of diabetes. I have four decades of education and experience of living with diabetes, if I can share my knowledge with you, then you too, will have the benefit of four decades of learning; acquired in the few hours that it takes to read my book.

My approach to diabetes has changed at various times in my life and I have struggled to manage my diabetes, rebelling at certain points in my life against my diabetes in negative ways. At other times I have been the most compliant patient you could hope to meet. I have made mistakes but I have always been looking for the best coping strategy at that point in my life. I have made many decisions about my diabetes – some excellent and others not so good. When you read this you will find strategies that may help you on your own personal journey with type 1 diabetes, some will be strategies that you might adopt, others may be strategies that you might want to avoid. Both of these outcomes contain knowledge well gained as you have learned something from my experiences.

CHAPTER TWO

DIAGNOSIS

In July of 1977, when I was just five years old, I was on a family holiday in Scotland with my older brother, Mum and Dad. I had just completed my first year at school. We had been away for a few days when I developed a raging thirst that just could not be quenched; we later learned that the lemonade I was drinking by the pint was not helping because it was loaded with sugar, making the problem worse. Not surprisingly I was peeing for England and, by all accounts, its entire population, I was so tired that if I was not drinking or peeing I was sleeping. I was taken to a local doctor for an emergency consultation and I was diagnosed with – a throat infection.

Within 24 hours my 'throat infection' was so bad that my breathing was now rapid and shallow; body fat was visibly falling off of me; my tongue was coated by a thick dry white substance, which was causing it to stick to the roof of my mouth; my fingers looked like I had sat in a bath for hours; and I had severe abdominal pain. Did I mention that I was peeing for the entire planet and had an incredible, insatiable thirst? An emergency doctor was called and he insisted that I should be admitted to hospital immediately. He told my parents that they did not have enough time to wait for an ambulance and that they should stop for nothing. I have no recollection of this journey but it happened in the early hours of the morning, I understand that my father drove at high speed passing through red traffic lights and junctions without hesitation. Within minutes of arriving at hospital I was diagnosed with type 1 diabetes and severe Diabetic Ketoacidosis (DKA) and insulin therapy was started. However, because my nervous system had become so severely depressed by the DKA and dehydration, I slipped into a coma shortly after arriving. It took 48 hours of insulin therapy and intravenous rehydration therapy before I came back from that coma.

My Mum, Dad and brother had a very steep learning curve over the next two weeks so that I could be discharged from hospital into their care. They were learning to count carbohydrates and calculate insulin doses, which was more difficult back then because some insulin was at 40 percent strength and some was at 80 percent. Consequently, you had to have the correct insulin and syringe for the strength administered. I remember being taken out of the hospital for a few hours by Mum and Dad and walked into the local town just before lunch time, so that my blood glucose levels would fall and I would become hypoglycaemic. Of course, Mum and Dad had to learn how to deal with this too. We all had to learn how to measure glucose levels, which was an arcane art involving mixing five drops of urine with ten drops of fresh water in a test tube. Then we added a Clinitest tablet, which would fizz up and change colour – blue meant that there was no glucose in the urine and orange meant that there were excessive amounts. I now know that this is a Benedict's reducing sugars reaction and has little value in managing diabetes, but that was all we had as routine blood glucose testing was still some years away.

At the age of seven I went to a summer camp for children with diabetes where I learned to administer my own injections. These days injections are quite simple, but then we had to perform complex calculations to work out the number of units required. We also had to sterilise heavy glass syringes and needles as they were not disposable; we reused them many times, storing them in a small vial of surgical spirit between injections and pushing a small wire brush down the needle to clean the aperture of the needle. The other important thing that I learned at camp was how other children and adults were dealing with diabetes in an everyday context, in other words, how to have the confidence to live a 'normal' life.

A second key event happened that year when I had a minor routine operation on my nose. I was taken into hospital the day before surgery was scheduled. Later that night I was awakened by a nurse who insisted that I drink a glass of milk because I was not going to be having my insulin the next morning because it would affect the anaesthetic. I must have sounded like a very precocious seven-year-old when I refused the milk and demanded to be allowed to use the phone, informing the nurse that I needed my insulin and the doctor was going to kill me if he did not allow me to have my insulin. Needless to say, I was confined to my bed and refused access to the phone. I did not manage to sleep again that night. When I was taken to the operating theatre the next morning they still insisted that I could not have insulin.

After coming around from the anaesthetic I was in severe Diabetic Ketoacidosis (DKA), which results only from a severe lack of insulin. This means that I had the same symptoms that I originally presented with at the age of five; although I was not yet in a coma. I now understand that not only did I need the normal insulin dose, but I should have been given additional rapid-acting insulin, such as existed in 1979. This was because my blood glucose levels were almost certainly going to rise as a result of the stress hormones (including adrenaline and cortisol) that were being released. These hormones make you resistant to insulin, if I had consumed that milk the situation would have been worse since milk is a rich source of sugar (lactose). My luck changed when my mum, who was told that she could not visit me that day, came to the hospital in the early evening. I was about 12 hours post surgery, and it had been 36 hours since my last insulin dose. Mum took control of the situation, raising the endocrinology consultant on the phone, and she was able to get an emergency prescription of insulin so that my life could be saved.

However, I am thankful for the medical professionals who displayed amazing levels of incompetence with respect to diabetes during my formative years, because when I left the hospital the morning after surgery I decided that I was never going to leave my healthcare in the hands of medical professionals again. Aged just seven years old I began to read everything that I could find about diabetes. I do still go to the doctor if I am unwell, although I am pleased to say that this happens rarely, and I do attend regular diabetes clinic appointments. The difference is that I now recognise that I am the expert on my diabetes and that medical care and prescriptions require my consent. I suspect that my medical team may hate me because I am the difficult customer with the awkward questions. I read the research papers and, when I cannot find the answers, I ask my very understanding and infinitely patient consultant, but he usually cannot answer them either!

TIP

You live with diabetes 24 hours a day, 7 days a week, 52 weeks a year. It is your gift to become an expert in your own health and to learn the steps that you need to take to do the very best for your own health. You will learn new things every day; some of these lessons you will relearn again and again and sometimes they are new lessons. These lessons are always useful in helping me to reflect on the strategies that serve me best.

As a result of my vast experience with diabetes I have helped many people over the years to understand their diabetes or take positive actions to manage their diabetes, rather than being controlled by this potentially devastating disorder. I have invested considerable time in coaching adults, children, and parents. I have seen that with some coaching, people go on to do amazing things, maybe in spite of or perhaps because they have diabetes.

If you have diabetes you will not lead an ordinary life. As a person with diabetes your life will be filled with many extras: extra medical care and consultations, extra vigilance and monitoring of your own health, extra blood tests, extra care with respect to your diet, in fact, extra preparation in everything that you do. Some people might view the added dimensions as burdens, but, from my own perspective, this simply means that my life is exceptional, and only a small adjustment is required to make it extraordinary. I know that this sounds clichéd, but before you dismiss the notion, please consider that because you have type 1 diabetes, you have a special and powerful gift. You can give someone less fortunate than you the gift of life almost without cost and certainly without pain. Sounds too good to be true, doesn't it?

If you had been diagnosed with diabetes before 1922 you would have died, there was no way to treat diabetes – insulin had not yet been isolated and purified. Today, people are still dying in some parts of the world because they cannot afford access to insulin. I urge everybody who is taking insulin to get in touch with the Insulin Dependant Diabetes Trust, as they send insulin that is nearing its expiry date to communities in India. In that country insulin is so expensive that families are forced to choose between the family eating or their relatives having the insulin they need to stay alive; unfortunately, relatives with diabetes often lose out with devastating results. They die. The Insulin Dependant Diabetes Trust distributes insulin for free in these communities. However, they need insulin to do this, and as a diabetic, you have a unique gift. For the cost of an envelope and a stamp every couple of months you can save lives by sending your insulin that is nearing its expiry date. In fact, before you continue reading this book, go and check the stocks of insulin that are building up in your fridge and get the old spare bottle/penfill/pre-filled pen and put it in the envelope immediately. STOP and do it NOW – take that action and remember to post the insulin.

The need is for these items:

- Insulin that is no longer needed, unopened, and in date (with at least 3 months left to the expiry date)

- Syringes, lancets and needles

- Glucose test strips

Please help if you can by sending the supplies you do not need to this address:

Insulin Dependent Diabetes Trust, PO Box 294, Northamptom NN1 4XS; Tel: 01604 622837; e-mail: insulin@iddtinternational.org

**THANK YOU,
YOU WILL HELP PEOPLE TO STAY ALIVE!**

Just take a moment to reflect upon how incredible it is that with the tiny effort of walking to the fridge and the post box, at the cost of only an envelope and a stamp, you just saved the life of a complete stranger. Congratulations! You are an extraordinary person doing extraordinary things. How many of your friends and colleagues can say that they saved the life of somebody who lives thousands of miles away today? Your diabetes has given you an incredible opportunity.

I am certain that everybody with diabetes has experienced, and probably continues to experience, a multitude of advice from people who know little or nothing about living with diabetes. This advice will be about the things that you can or cannot do; some of it comes from well-meaning friends and relatives, some comes from medical professionals. Let's set the record straight here – you can do anything that you want. Sir Steve Redgrave achieved five gold medals in four consecutive Olympic games for rowing, but did you realise that he was diagnosed with diabetes between his third and fourth Olympic games? Five Olympic gold medals is an incredible achievement even before you consider that he has diabetes! Did Sir Steve Redgrave win that medal by doubting that he could do it? Did he believe that his diabetes would prevent his success? I know that the cynics out there will be saying it is OK for him as he was already famous and successful and he could afford the best care. The good news is that, if you live in the UK, you can get access to the same world-class team of experts on diabetes and exercise through the NHS. Your GP can refer you to the team, and information about them can be found at www.runsweet.org or type Dr Ian Gallen into a search engine. Even if you do not live in the UK, please do check the website as it is a fantastic resource, and exercise is a loose term here, since it covers everything from children playing to Olympic-standard rowing and just about anything in between.

My attitude is never ever to say I cannot do that because I am diabetic. Instead, I ask different questions: How can I do that? What preparation and/or changes to my diabetes care do I need to make to make sure that I can do that? Remember that your mind is always right; if you say I cannot do something, you are right as you will not be able to do it. Instead ask yourself – how can I do that? Who can I ask, copy, or learn from? Do I know anybody who can help me with this?

You will find that suddenly new resources are available, and you will achieve things that other people have considered impossible. This is true of everything in life, so why should diabetes be any different? To demonstrate this point I will be joining nineteen other people with type 1 diabetes and climbing Mount Kilimanjaro in June 2014. Mount Kilimanjaro is a challenging environment for everybody, but for somebody with type 1 diabetes there are additional challenges to cope with. We each have our own reasons for doing this trip, but collectively we are demonstrating to the world that diabetes is not a barrier to achieving your dreams, whatever they may be.

Some years ago I was fortunate enough to attend some fantastic nutrition lectures that were given by Dr Wyndham Boobier at the University of Glamorgan (these were not related to diabetes, but to nutrition in general). The content of the lectures has always remained with me, but the headline that I will always remember was the opening sentence of the opening lecture. Dr Boobier said, in front of a packed lecture theatre. "You have a choice: if you are lucky enough to live to be 65 years old, you can live in an old people's home; you can have arthritis, cancer, and incontinence, or you can be like me; I am going to celebrate my 80th birthday by going surfing. The choice is yours, pissing yourself at 65 or surfing at 80, what is it going to be?" Dr Boobier spoke in some detail over a series of lectures about the right nutrition, and these details will be an essential part of his journey to that 80th birthday party. But in my opinion just as important is his amazingly positive and passionate attitude to life.

I am going to summarise this section with five key quotes that define my own philosophy of living with diabetes:

- *"I decided early on that diabetes was going to live with me, not me live with diabetes."* Sir Steven Redgrave.

- *"There is no reason why you cannot achieve your dreams but it does take a lot of practice and patience to work out the right routine."* Sir Steven Redgrave.

- *"The quality of your life is a reflection of the quality of the questions that you ask."* Anthony Robbins

- *"The patient with diabetes who knows the most about diabetes, lives the longest."* Elliot P Joslin (1922)

- *"Education leads to empowerment."* Paul Coker

CHAPTER THREE

THE BASICS AND BEYOND

Type 1 diabetes cannot be prevented and it is not caused by lifestyle choices. At the present time we do not understand why the body's own immune system turns upon the insulin producing cells in the pancreas. If you have type 1 diabetes (please forgive me for asking this question) but would you know what undiagnosed type 1 diabetes looks like? What symptoms does someone with undiagnosed type 1 diabetes have? Diabetes UK is currently running a fantastic advertising campaign, which describes the presentation of type 1 diabetes in what they call the 4 T's:

- **Tired** – tired all of the time

- **Thirsty** – thirsty all of the time, often even as soon as a drink is finished

- **Thinner** – sudden weight loss

- **Toilet** – weeing a lot

If you see these symptoms in a loved one get them to a doctor immediately and demand that the doctor performs a very simple, painless, quick and cheap urine test to check for glucose in the urine. Doctors can be reluctant to do this test but, in all honesty, it takes about 30 seconds to do and costs just a few pennies. It can be performed in the doctor's surgery, with no need for any laboratory results, and the results are instantaneous.

I make no apology for preaching the signs of diabetes to people who are already knowledgeable in diabetes, I hear too many tales of children being admitted to hospital with Diabetic Ketoacidosis when they, displaying all the signs of diabetes, have been seeing their family doctor for the last few weeks. I understand that many of you have already seen all of these symptoms and would recognise diabetes in an instant, but, if just one person reads this and recognises undiagnosed diabetes in a friend or relative, then these words are invaluable.

Most people have heard of diabetes, but for most the only experience they have of diabetes is with type 2 diabetes, so let us talk a little about type 2 diabetes here. Type 2 diabetes accounts for about 90 percent of all cases worldwide. In the UK, this means there are about four million people with type 2 diabetes as of 2013. Type 2 diabetes shares some common features with type 1 diabetes, this causes a great deal of confusion with both the general public and the medical community. Type 2 diabetes is often associated with lifestyle choices. The typical patient with type 2 diabetes is over 40 years old, overweight, and has a sedentary lifestyle. There is growing evidence that, for many people, type 2 diabetes can be reversed by changing to a healthier lifestyle. I apologise here to all people with type 2 diabetes who don't fit this pattern, but you are the exception that proves the rule.

People with type 2 diabetes may still produce insulin, but the effectiveness of their insulin is impaired, or they cannot produce enough insulin. Initially treatment is usually to lose some weight, to take regular exercise and to modify their diet, substituting high-fat, simple carbohydrates for low-fat, complex carbohydrates. If this is not sufficient to effect blood glucose management tablets may be prescribed which will help the cells to use the insulin that they have more efficiently or will boost insulin production. To confuse matters some people with type 2 diabetes can end up on insulin injections. However, even if they are using insulin, they do not have type 1 diabetes, as the immune system has little involvement in the causes and presentation of type 2 diabetes. Most importantly, the onset of type 2 diabetes is slow and insidious, taking many years to develop and those affected often don't realise that they have it. They have a very slow and gradual increase in blood glucose levels, which makes them feel gradually more tired and lethargic. In general, people often sadly decide this is because they are getting older, therefore, they spend years walking around with undiagnosed and untreated type 2 diabetes, suffering terrible consequences to their own health.

Type 1 diabetes is completely different and it can be diagnosed at any age. Although it is most commonly diagnosed in young people, the most common age being twelve years of age. There is limited data informing us how long it takes for the immune system to destroy the insulin-producing cells which will lead to type 1 diabetes; however, some researchers think it can take as little as six months. The reduction in the population of insulin-producing cells will lead to gradually increased blood glucose levels. The full effects of type 1 diabetes are not normally visible until the population of these cells drops to 30 percent of normal or less. When this happens it is like falling from a cliff edge: Blood glucose levels will rise suddenly, and the symptoms of type 1 diabetes will happen very quickly indeed.

In my own case over a four-day period, I went from being apparently healthy to being in a coma caused by high blood glucose levels. The inability to produce insulin is not compatible with life and the only treatment that is available for people with type 1 diabetes is to give insulin, either by injection or by using an insulin pump. To the best of my knowledge, it is not common for pumps to be given to patients at the time of diagnosis, although this will change in time. Insulin must be taken as an injection or delivered through a cannula, because it is a protein and would be digested by the acids in the stomach, meaning that it would never get to be active and transported in the blood where it is required. A few years ago a system of inhaling insulin was developed, similar to a very large asthma pump, and it did briefly become available. But the system was hindered by the large size of the delivery mechanism and an inability to fine tune the insulin dose, and I believe has now been withdrawn.

Most people know that there is a relationship between diabetes and insulin, anybody with type 1 diabetes is acutely aware just how important insulin is – but what is it? How does insulin work? Why can't we take a shot of insulin four times a day, and then carry on regardless? Why do many people hear the word diabetes and immediately assume that means that you cannot eat sugar?

To answer these questions properly we first need to look at insulin production and use in people who don't have diabetes. It is essential that we understand that maintenance of normal blood glucose levels are essential to the optimal functioning of every cell in the body, and that the body invests a huge amount of effort to make sure that the blood glucose levels remain within a target range at all times. There are a number of mechanisms that the body uses to control blood glucose levels, and insulin is an integral part of the process. Insulin is required at all times, even when we are not eating or drinking carbohydrates.

Insulin is a protein formed from 51 amino acids and, when used for therapeutic purposes, it is genetically engineered and manufactured to ensure that we have the supplies that we need in the purest form possible. In addition to its classification as a protein, insulin is a hormone because it is released into the blood for circulation and used widely throughout the body. Like most hormones, its production and release is controlled by part of the brain called the hypothalamus.

It is worth taking a few minutes here to describe in detail our cells, which are the building blocks of our bodies. The cell is a distinct unit, and the human body is made up of millions of them. Each cell maintains its own unique internal environment that is distinctly different from the outside of the cell, and the cell wall (also known as the cell or plasma membrane) is responsible for maintaining this environment. The very special structure of the cell membrane makes it selectively permeable, meaning that some things can get into the cell whilst others get out, but almost always in response to the cells needs, relative to both its internal and external environment. Some essential substances need the assistance of a transport mechanism to cross the cell membrane. Specifically, in the case of diabetes, the cell membrane isn't permeable to glucose (except for certain neural cells and the germinal epithelia of the reproductive system) and insulin is required to act as a key which binds to the cell membrane and allows glucose to pass from the blood to the inside of the cell. The glucose is used by special structures inside the cell called mitochondria, which provide power to the cell. Without insulin, the concentration of glucose in the blood rises to dangerously high levels whilst the cells are starved of the essential fuel that they need to live. The majority of glucose available to most of us comes from the carbohydrates that we eat in our diets, which gives us the basis for people with type 1 diabetes and some people with type 2 diabetes to give insulin at or near meal times.

However, insulin does much more than allow glucose to cross the cell membrane. There is a limit to the amount of glucose that our cells can use at any one time and, in the event of an excess of glucose, the body stores it for later use in a variety of ways, and insulin is an essential conduit in this storage system. The first response to an excess of glucose in the blood is to store it and, in the presence of insulin, glucose gets converted to a chemical called glycogen, which is stored in the liver and muscle cells. It is converted back to glucose between meals when the blood glucose levels start to drop or when exercise is undertaken. This provides an important buffering system for the blood glucose levels, if they fall too low insulin shock or hypoglycaemia occurs, remember that the operation of the central nervous system is almost entirely dependant upon the availability of adequate levels of plasma glucose.

TIP

Insulin is classified as both a protein and a hormone. Its primary function is to act as a key that binds to the cell walls, allowing fuel to enter the cells.

The volume of insulin required varies from moment to moment in people with and without diabetes. The biggest challenge for people with type 1 diabetes is making exactly the right amount of active insulin available at exactly the right time given the internal and external environments of the individual cells and the body as a whole.

Too much insulin causes low blood glucose levels and is the cause of hypoglycaemia; untreated hypoglycaemia is a life-threatening medical emergency. Not enough insulin leads to high blood glucose levels and can lead to a life-threatening medical emergency called Diabetic Ketoacidosis.

The liver is able to increase its mass by about five to six percent and the muscles by about two to three percent in the right circumstances, so that they can store glycogen (a form of glucose). When these boundaries are reached insulin is used to convert excess glucose into fatty acids, triglycerides and lipoproteins, which are then packaged and stored as adipose tissue (fat). In times of starvation little insulin is available and an enzyme called hormone sensitive lipase releases triglycerides from adipose tissue, and the cycle is reversed until glucose is made available to the cells via the blood again, provided that blood glucose levels remain stable.

In diabetes as the cells are starved of fuel by the lack of insulin the same thing happens and the body is stripped of its fat, and the plasma levels of lipids increase due to a lack of insulin (cholesterol, fatty acids, and triglycerides). If this is allowed to happen over extended periods of time the increased plasma levels are thought to cause trauma to the cardiovascular system. In type 1 diabetes this is typically the microvessels in the eyes, kidneys, and heart, leading respectively to retinopathy, renal failure, and heart disease – which are common long-term consequences of diabetes. It is worth mentioning that some people choose to manage their weight at low levels by giving suboptimal levels of insulin, and this is a form of anorexia and is extremely dangerous to one's health in the short and long term. In the long term, the risk is to the cardiovascular system and in the immediate term, the risk is of Diabetic Ketoacidosis, which is a life-threatening medical emergency.

Insulin increases the permeability of the cell membrane to amino acids (the building blocks of protein) and also increases the uptake of potassium and phosphate ions. This is important in allowing the cell to construct the environment and electrical charge that it needs to operate. Perhaps even more important is that insulin plays a role in RNA (ribonucleic acid) translation, which is an intermediate step in cell replication and in the transcription of (duplicating) DNA (deoxyribonucleic acid). This is quite a profound revelation and could potentially lead to cell lines that are damaged by inadequate insulin availability, which could affect us today and in the future, if these damaged cells are viable and go on to replicate.

As we have seen, insulin is a complex multifaceted substance which serves essential roles in the metabolism of carbohydrates, fats, and proteins. Insulin also works in concert with other hormones to ensure that blood glucose remains stable. Insulin is produced in the pancreas by the islets of Langerhans' Beta cells, its principal role is to lower blood glucose levels. Insulin activity peaks about six minutes after it is released, within fifteen minutes of secretion, it is inactive. When blood glucose levels are falling too fast or too low, the pancreas produces another hormone called glucagon, which promotes the breakdown of glycogen from the liver and muscle cells to raise blood glucose levels. Only very small amounts of glucagon have a huge effect on raising blood glucose levels because of the cascade effect that it has at each of its biochemical changes, which it goes through to make glucose available. Glucagon reaches its peak activity in about three minutes and is inactive after about eight to ten minutes. Another hormone released by the pancreas called somatotropin inhibits the action of both insulin and glucagon to ensure that blood glucose remains in range. Innately produced insulin peaks in activity after just six minutes. Suddenly, we can see why people with diabetes who use insulin are at risk of hypoglycaemia, when our injected insulin has an action profile of at least four hours instead of fifteen minutes.

People with diabetes who use insulin can eat carbohydrates, fats and proteins, provided that they compensate appropriately with insulin. The volume of insulin and timing of a dose need careful consideration and some appreciation of environmental conditions is essential. The level of activity over the coming hours must be planned if blood glucose levels are to remain in target. To explain this a little more let's take the example of eating a pizza and how it can be a complicated affair. The base is usually made of a bread-like, wheat-flour mix that is covered with tomato, topped with cheese, a few herbs and any other toppings that appeal. We think it sounds fairly safe if a little greasy, so why is it that so many people struggle to get their dose of insulin just right after eating it? The answer is that the high-fat content of the pizza delays the absorption of carbohydrates because it takes the gut longer to digest fats than pure carbohydrates. In a pizza, fats and carbohydrates are bound together, and therefore, the gut must break the fats and carbohydrates apart, which takes some time and effort. People with diabetes often find that in the hours following eating a pizza that their blood glucose level rise to relatively high levels, I know many people who use an insulin pump which has a biphasic or dual wave/multi-wave, insulin delivery system and they call it the pizza setting for this very reason.

Just in case these factors are not complex enough, there are a number of other issues which will promote insulin absorption. These might include very hot weather, very cold weather and exercise. Conversely stress and caffeine make me resistant to insulin and, like many people with diabetes, the natural release of cortisol in the early hours of the morning (a normal part of the sleep-wake cycle) makes me resistant to insulin until mid-morning. Each of these stressors on my system needs to be accommodated in my insulin dose and in the timings of my insulin delivery.

We are now starting to understand that giving a shot of insulin is never a straightforward process. There are so many variables that will impact upon how well the insulin is absorbed or not and, for much of the time, we are not consciously aware of small day-to-day changes that may be affecting our ability to use insulin.

The amount of insulin that we need is not constant. We commonly observe that there are variations in our insulin needs, depending on many different influences. Everything from the weather to the amount of exercise we have done or are going to do has an influence on blood glucose levels and the amount of insulin we need. My own experience is that I need less insulin in hot weather and more in cold weather. I don't yet understand the reason for this: Is it the influence of temperature on my body? Is it when the sun is shining and it is hot that I am more physically active?

Exercise is probably one of the best things that you can do to manage your diabetes, but it is also one of the biggest challenges to maintaining blood glucose levels that we face. Increased levels of activity allow some cells and receptors in the muscles to use glucose without requiring insulin as a conduit. This is great for lowering blood glucose levels and improving insulin sensitivity; however, it means that insulin users must be aware of this and must make compensations in the amount of insulin they have on board before they exercise. The term 'exercise' here could mean anything from playing on the swings in the park to running a half marathon, or as in the case of Sir Steven Redgrave, who has diabetes, winning gold medals for rowing in the Olympics.

Many things influence blood glucose levels and the amount of insulin required. The table below gives a simple view of some of the common factors which influence blood glucose levels:

Lowers Blood Glucose Levels	Raises Blood Glucose Levels
Insulin	Carbohydrates
Exercise	Glycogen
Stress	Infection and Illness
Illness (sometimes)	Caffeine
Some Prescription Medications	Cortisol
	Adrenaline (Epinephrine)
Alcohol	Stress
	Anaerobic Exercise
	Menstrual Cycle

We have spent a lot of time talking about insulin and its role in maintaining stable blood glucose. Why do blood glucose levels need to be maintained so well? Glucose is the energy that our cells need in order to survive and carry out normal functions. When glucose is not available the cells are starved of fuel, the very survival of those cells is threatened. When insulin is not available, and the body's glucose cannot cross the cell membrane, the cells are starving in a sea of plenty. The distress signals from these cells instigates a survival mechanism in the body to release glucose from the liver and muscles. This response adds glucose to the blood, but that glucose still cannot be used, and the concentration of glucose in the blood climbs again. The cells are still starved of fuel and the body switches over to burning fat as a fuel source (fats are essentially a store of carbohydrates and water). The burning of fat releases high volumes of glucose into the blood, but once again without insulin, the glucose is unable to cross the plasma membrane and the cells continue to be starved of fuel whilst the concentration of glucose in the blood continues to climb. Eventually, the body starts to convert proteins into glucose as an emergency energy source, which further increases blood glucose concentrations, but still the blood glucose cannot fuel the cells. The blood is now loaded with excessively high concentrations of glucose and, in an attempt to restore the blood glucose concentration, the kidneys allow glucose to be lost in the urine, which causes damage to the kidneys. As the kidneys try to bring the blood glucose concentrations down they produce masses of urine as a transport conduit for the excess glucose and you become excessively thirsty in an attempt to maintain the correct water volume in your body.

The picture we have now is of somebody who is massively dehydrated, has lost most of the body's fat, is peeing more than he or she is able to drink and is drinking excessively with a thirst that cannot be quenched. As if this picture was not bad enough the by-product of the body eating its own protein stores for conversion to glucose is a toxic acid called a ketone body, which gets transported in the blood. Unfortunately, the blood has only a minimal tolerance for changes in its acid/alkalis balance and very quickly the acidity of the blood rises. At this point, the body reacts urgently and shallow rapid breathing starts in order to bring carbon dioxide into the system to buffer this acidity. This situation, which is called Diabetic Ketoacidosis (DKA), cannot be reversed until sufficient insulin is available and, left untreated, DKA will lead to coma and death very quickly. DKA is a medical emergency and must be treated with insulin and intravenous fluids to restore normal function of the central nervous system.

Surely, the alternative is to give lots of insulin so that DKA can never happen. Right? Wrong. Too much insulin causes its own problems. In the presence of insulin, the body is unable to convert the glucose stores in the liver and muscles, and too much insulin leads to a low blood glucose level, which is known as hypoglycaemia (or hypo for short). I cannot tell you what a hypo looks like from the outside because I have never seen one since I have only been at the receiving end. For me, and I understand this is quite common, the symptoms of a hypo can vary enormously from episode to episode, sometimes with early warning systems like tingling in the hands or lips. Sometimes with profuse sweating, other times with irritability or becoming extremely friendly and talking a lot. At times there are no symptoms at all. I am led to believe that, to an observer, a person suffering a hypo looks a lot like a drunk. The treatment for a hypo is to take glucose preferably in the form of dextrose which is absorbed readily and quickly and, in my experience, prevents overtreatment of the hypo and the subsequent high blood glucose level.

You might be forgiven for thinking that hypoglycaemia is the lesser of the two evils, but one of my friends crashed his car off of the road and into a tree whilst driving when hypoglycaemia struck him suddenly. He survived the crash, but fractured his arm, suffered burns on his face from the airbag, and lost his driving licence on medical grounds. It is conservatively estimated by some researchers that up to six percent of deaths in people with type 1 diabetes are caused by night time hypoglycaemia. The hypothesis is that people sleep through a hypo, the subsequent release of adrenaline and cortisol, places a huge stress on the heart as adrenaline and cortisol are released to compensate for low blood glucose levels, leading to a heart attack. You might be forgiven for thinking this only happens to older people, but unfortunately, it happens in children too.

Perhaps another solution might be to run blood glucose levels a little high, not high enough to cause DKA, but above normal levels so that you prevent a hypo. Sounds great doesn't it? Well, just like everything else in diabetes, it is never quite that simple. Running blood glucose levels at higher levels increases the chances of long-term complications or secondary symptoms of diabetes. The Diabetes Control & Complications Trial (DCCT) 1992 demonstrates that, for every 10 percent decrease in our long-term blood glucose measurement through a test called the HbA1c, there is a 35 percent decrease in the risk of developing retinopathy. Retinopathy is a diabetic eye disease and is the leading cause of blindness in the working-age population in both the USA and the UK. The answer is that we must find ways to maintain near normal good glucose levels at all times to protect our own health.

TIP

The best way that people with type 1 diabetes can protect their health is to maintain blood glucose levels as near to normal as possible. The technical name for this is euglycemia and acquiring and maintaining it is the holy grail of diabetes management.

I have helped many parents of newly diagnosed children come to deal with diabetes in their lives. I commonly see that these parents are so frightened by the consequences they have learned about high blood glucose levels that they give their children so much insulin that these children spend a lot of time with low blood glucose levels. Low blood glucose levels are dangerous and should be avoided. Six out of every hundred people with diabetes, who are otherwise healthy, will die as a result of low blood glucose levels. Don't let it be you or the one you love. Learn how to recognise a hypo – treat it and minimise the amount of times that it happens.

I would not wish a low blood glucose level on anybody. I usually feel disorientated and confused, and I get disturbances in my vision. If they happen at night, I can wake up drenched in sweat, trembling, and unable to reach out to my bedside table to reach for my glucose, which is only an arm's length away. Like many people with type 1 diabetes, I hate being hypo and will go to extreme lengths to avoid it.

CHAPTER FOUR

DIABETES MANAGEMENT IS EMOTIONAL

You might be surprised to learn my first, and most effective tool, in managing my diabetes is not about measuring blood glucose levels, or giving a bolus of insulin, or measuring carbohydrates, or testing my basal insulin rates. Taking appropriate insulin at the right time is essential, but the most effective and powerful tool that I have in managing my diabetes is the language that I use, because it changes my perception of diabetes, and this empowers me to make the best choices at any given time.

When I was diagnosed, home blood glucose monitoring was yet to be developed. I used to measure the content of glucose in my urine with an alchemy kit, applying five droplets of urine to ten droplets of water and adding a Clinitest tablet to the mix. This mixture would bubble and fizz and turn different colours – blue meant no glucose present, green a small amount and orange was a lot of glucose. This was always called a urine test and, in the brain of a young child, I could either pass the test (blue) or fail (orange). I remember that my mother used to make some judgements about whether I had been controlling my diabetes based upon those results. I also remember that on occasions when there were cakes and sweets I might be allowed some if I 'passed' my urine test. On many occasions I purposely neglected to add the urine so that I would pass the test. On other occasions, when complacency had set in, instead of measuring the doses of water and urine with a pipette I would guesstimate it by eye. It is, therefore, obvious that for me at least using the words 'urine test' held negative connotations, and, for this reason, I will only ever refer to measuring blood glucose levels. You can neither fail or pass a blood glucose measurement and you can only gather data which will empower you to make focused decisions on your diabetes management.

Why is using the right language important to managing diabetes? Words are powerful tools and are used to convey information; often words have emotional attachments and they will vary from individual to individual. I am sure that we can all think of words that make us smile, cringe, or laugh out loud. If you get a group of seven-year-old children together and say a word like 'bum', they will soon start to laugh; conversely, if you say words like 'tidy your room', the response is likely to be quite different. I use these examples to demonstrate the point, but we can equally attach positive and negative emotions to terms that we use to describe diabetes and the tools that we use to manage the condition. Terms like hospital check-up must be avoided at all costs, instead use terms like 'my diabetes consultation', and you will suddenly find that you are empowered to take the lead role in your diabetes consultation.

We really must choose our words carefully; they define not only who we are and the actions that we take, but they also define who others think we are. To give you an idea about the power of words, tomorrow when you meet people, ask them how they are. I can guarantee you that most responses will be 'not too bad' or 'fine'. Who in their right mind would settle for 'not too bad'? If your standards of how you are feeling today are 'not too bad', also known as 'I feel bad, but I have felt worse', then your day, week, month, year, decade or life is going to be bad because you are focusing on feeling bad. You really do get more of what you focus on. Tomorrow, when somebody asks you how you are, I want you to run a little exercise in your mind before you answer. Remember that no matter if your blood glucose levels are high or you are recovering from the worst hypo that you have had this year, in the last 24 hours you have done something absolutely amazing – you have survived another day with diabetes, and you have beaten the odds. The inability to produce insulin is not consistent with life, and, less than 100 years ago, an insulin injection would have been a miracle. You are amazing and you should be celebrated as a hero; you are beating the odds and setting new standards. Now that you realise that you are a truly outstanding person, who has done incredible and amazing things to survive the last 24 hours how are you feeling today? Did you say outstanding, fantastic, amazing, incredible or grateful? If not, why not? What stories are you telling yourself which stop you from feeling amazing?

TIP

Choose the language that empowers you in respect to your diabetes. Avoid terms like "blood glucose test", which can have negative connotations, instead measure your blood glucose levels and make decisions about the strategies you are going to use based upon that information. If you are looking after young children with diabetes, encourage them to be a part of that decision.

I am rewarded every time I am empowered to make decisions about my diabetes, because I can either continue to feel fantastic, or I can take the appropriate steps so that I feel brilliant again very quickly.

Join a support network and manage the support you get at home

I encourage anybody living with diabetes to join in the various online support networks. There are many of them and you will find that common questions and themes are being discussed in all of them. My favourite support group is without a doubt the insulin pumpers blog site, but there are many Facebook groups that offer great discussion forums. I have included a full section on useful resources for people with type 1 diabetes at the end of this book.

Developing a support network around you is one of the most useful tools that you will ever have in managing your diabetes. Over the years I have lost count of the number of times well-meaning friends and relatives have made me feel like they are judging me because of how I manage my diabetes. In doing research for this book, I found a fantastic article on www.diabetesdaily.com and my thanks go to Ginger Viera for allowing me to use her words here on this matter:

NON-DIABETIC'S GUIDE TO HELPING LOVED ONES WITH DIABETES

"Whether you're a brother, mother, aunt, boyfriend, wife or best friend, knowing how to support the people in your life who live with diabetes isn't all that easy. In fact, it can be very tricky. Mostly, because:

We all have different needs when it comes to the kind of support we want in diabetes.

You, as the person who loves us, really want to make sure we're safe and healthy, and sometimes that might come off as overbearing or controlling or nosey...but really, you just really love us.

We don't always behave the most wonderfully when we're having a high blood sugar or a low blood sugar. And while we can't always control that behaviour, it does make communication a lot harder for you, the person who loves us.

To help you be the best support system you can possibly be for the person in your life with diabetes, here are a few tips:

Ask us what we need. Personally, I don't need someone to remind me to check my blood sugar or help me count my carbohydrates. That would irritate me. On the other hand, it is incredibly helpful when my boyfriend reminds me to take my Lantus before bed, and I sincerely appreciate when he asks me what my blood sugar is after I check. To me, that's great support. I want him to know what my blood sugar is so he can be aware of how my mental state is. For others, those things might drive them nuts. Giving us support we don't want isn't going to help; in fact, it might lead us to blocking you out of our diabetes management altogether. Let us tell you, in our own words, how you can support us.

Please don't lecture us. Telling an adult with diabetes what we should or should not be doing is only appropriate when we've asked for your insight. Telling us that we shouldn't be eating that or shouldn't be drinking this comes from your heart, we know, but 99% of the time, those lecture-like comments from you are going to come off as controlling. To add to it, we are in-charge of what we put in our bodies. If we choose to make less-than-healthy decisions, that is our responsibility. Sometimes you eat unhealthy things, too, right? If you are a parent, you will need to become more involved at times, sometimes incredibly involved on an hourly basis, but it's still best to strive for supportive collaboration rather than lecturing.

Be patient when our blood sugars are too low or too high. This one is really hard, because sometimes when we're having a low blood sugar, we seem more or less fine. We're making coherent decisions, we're moving our bodies normally–but inside, our brains are desperately begging for sugar in order to operate correctly. When our blood sugars are low, we literally do not have the fuel we need to think and communicate well, making it almost impossible to handle normal conversation. Instead of trying to talk to us, help us get glucose and don't expect anything else from us until our number has come back up within the next 15 to 30 minutes. When our blood sugars are high, we really want to curl into a ball and close our eyes. It doesn't feel good. Sometimes, it feels like a really quick bout of the flu (even when there are no ketones, and my blood sugar is barely over 200 mg/dL). To you, we might look fine because we can move and speak clearly, but we just don't feel right. And we need your compassionate patience. If our blood sugar is high, please think of us as someone who is sick with the flu for a short-period of time, until our number comes back down. Sometimes, a quick walk can help. Other times, lying on the couch and waiting is the best idea. Let us tell you.

When supporting and caring for children, diabetes brings a level of responsibility and daily management that is too much for a child to be expected to assume on their own. This means that being there, regularly, is crucial, but how you shape your presence and support can make all the difference in how that child grows up feeling and thinking about their diabetes. Helping to instill a habit (like checking blood sugars) versus nagging about the habit are very different. Focus on being a positive and encouraging part of their team, rather than someone whom they feel is always telling them what to do. Help engage them in their own diabetes management with questions, like, "So, your blood sugar is high. What do you think is the best way for us to handle this?" and help them think out loud about the next step, teaching them as you go and working together as a team.

In the end, we truly appreciate you. We do. We have no idea what it's like to live with, love, and watch someone we care about living with diabetes and not being able to truly know what they're going through. You want to take care of us, keep us safe, and help us live a happy, healthy life. Thank you! Just be sure to remember that what feels like support to you might not be the kind of support we're looking for. Ask us how you can be the best source of support in our lives with diabetes...but please, just don't ask when our blood sugars are low."

TIP

Your support network is essential to your health. Educate them well so that they provide you with the specific support mechanisms that you need. If you have not already done so, join one of the ever growing, online support groups for people with type 1 diabetes.

Manage Your Fear

'You can't do that, you have diabetes' is one of my prime motivators. When somebody tells me this, it is like a red flag to a bull. I have spent my whole life with people telling me things like you cannot walk around barefoot because you have diabetes and you could get an injury that wouldn't be noticeable (due to neurological damage and/or circulatory damage as a result of long-standing diabetes). Whilst I accept that this is a very real risk factor for people with diabetes, should I let them stop me from walking on the beach? This is very much a personal decision and must be based upon individual risk factors and your attitude to risk.

Personally, I have exhibited no evidence of neurological or circulatory defects in my feet yet, and to celebrate 36 years with type 1 diabetes one of my challenges was to do a fire walk, which involved walking barefoot across burning coals at 2000 degrees. It was a truly remarkable experience with 6,000 people behind me as a mutual support group. It taught me to manage my fears. It taught me that the limitations that we place on ourselves and allow others to place upon us are usually the boundaries of our existence, they are normally self-imposed, or we allow others to impose their beliefs upon us. During my fire walk my feet did not get burned or harmed in any way, in case you were wondering. The purpose of the fire walk is surprisingly not about walking on fire, but to teach us that when we rise above our self-inflicted boundaries and we elect to control our fears rather than let our fears control us, we can truly do things that are 'impossible'.

How many times have you been told that your diabetes is a barrier to doing something? How many times did that get you mad? How many times was the advice you received correct? What would you do if you did not have diabetes? Why is diabetes stopping you from doing that right now? It is true that there are some things that diabetes is an obstacle for but, the truth is, if we want anything badly enough, we will find a way to do it. The next time that you feel you cannot do something because you have diabetes, you need to find a role model, who has been through something similar or has a pushed the boundaries of diabetes beyond the normal expectations.

In almost every single aspect that I can think of the limitations that diabetes places upon you are the limitations that you place on yourself, or those that you consent to being placed upon you by others. I am certain that for every 'you cannot do that because you have diabetes', there is somebody who has done something similar. Famous examples of role models might include Gary Mabutt, who had a very successful career as a professional footballer, playing for England, even though he was diagnosed with type 1 diabetes in his late teens. Sir Steve Redgrave won gold medals at five consecutive Olympic Games even after he was diagnosed with diabetes.

Sometimes we need to look beyond the celebrity status for our role models, let me give you an example; Diana Maynard is a remarkable lady, she was diagnosed with type 1 diabetes at the age of 8. Her father had type 1 diabetes and so she grew up in a family where diabetes was the norm but also where diabetes had devastating consequences – Diana's father had severe and life limiting complications of diabetes. In fact Diana herself has complications caused by her diabetes which means that she has substantial loss of sight and she is classified as blind, and yet in spite of all of this to celebrate her 40th birthday Diana climbed Kilimanjaro. She regularly plays softball (in a sighted team) and she refuses to let her diabetes or the loss of her sight prevent her from doing things. As I wrote this chapter Diana was celebrating Christmas by climbing to Everest Base Camp. I find Diana's story absolutely inspirational, she overcomes her health and physical challenges by facing her fears and deciding to do things that others would consider too hard or even impossible. If you are ever told that you can't do something because you have diabetes just remember Diana, she climbs the world's highest mountains, she has diabetes and she is blind. What will your diabetes inspire you to do?

In preparing this book I interviewed Carol, the mother of a now teenaged girl called Michelle, who was diagnosed with type 1 diabetes when she was nine years old. Her local clinic was run by a consultant who believed that diabetes management was a 'one size fits all'. The consultant had obviously never lived a single day with diabetes or with somebody who had diabetes. The treatment protocol was very regimented and the story that Carol told me was of a regime that was more restricted than my own childhood experiences. Michelle's diabetes management plan was of a strict dietary regime, which left her so malnourished that she would cry in pain from the hunger. Her glucose control was poor and Carol and Michelle were led to believe that insulin doses could not be adjusted.

Michelle was on one injection each day. When Carol made enquiries about moving to two injections each day to improve Michelle's control and promote better long-term health, she was told it was completely unnecessary, and that all children regardless of age, size, and activity required exactly the same dose of insulin – which was one injection each day! Carol decided that this was not an acceptable treatment protocol for her daughter and withdrew her from the diabetes clinic, going it alone with a young child and no professional help or support. The local health authority investigated Carol and her husband, threatening to take Michelle into care because they were neglecting her medical needs. When Carol attended the meeting to determine if she was guilty of medical neglect, she provided detailed records of Michelle's insulin doses, carbohydrate intake, and blood glucose control. Clearly, she was not taking her to the hospital, but neglect was the furthest thing from her mind. She was just demanding a better standard of care for her daughter. The medical board agreed that Carol was taking good care of her daughter, and they referred Carol and Michelle to another clinic some distance from home.

At this point things improved for Michelle, but the distances involved in travelling were large, and it was becoming evident that multiple daily injections were not working for Michelle, since what she really needed was an insulin pump. Unfortunately the new clinic was unable to support a pump, and again, Carol became desperate to find the best care for her daughter. At this time Carol contacted an organisation called INPUT Diabetes who run a free advocacy service for people with diabetes (they assist people with diabetes in accessing appropriate medical technologies). With the help of INPUT Diabetes, and the amazing tenacity of Carol and Michelle, they found a clinic that could and would support them with an insulin pump! You would be forgiven for thinking that this story began 30 years ago when treatment was solely about keeping us alive, but the truth is that Michelle was only diagnosed with diabetes in 2006. I would like to say that this surprises me, but sadly, some medical practitioners are blatantly ignorant about type 1 diabetes. Fortunately for us, there are many more who are knowledgeable, but there are two things this tale reinforces for me:

- **The person with diabetes who knows the most about diabetes lives the longest**
- **It is your responsibility to define the standard of care you are willing to accept.**

Always remember to ask better questions if you want to improve the quality of your life and be inspired to live life to the fullest. What does this mean in practical terms? The reality is that you need to make some subtle, but powerful changes in your mindset. Instead of accepting that diabetes means you can't do something, you must ask yourself how you can do something even though you have diabetes. Let me give you an example; in October 2013, I ran my first half marathon. I decided early in my training programme that having a hypo during the event was not acceptable to me, and so, I asked the question: How can I run 13.1 miles and maintain a normal, stable blood glucose level? After a lot of research and even more training, I was able to complete the event; my blood glucose level was 8.2mmol/l (148mg/dL) at the start of the event and 7.0mmol/l (126mg/dL) at the end. I did not experience any hypos and I felt incredible throughout the whole event. I was able to do this because I was able to ask some great questions and I found some brilliant coaches. My success was in no small part built upon the strategies of at least five different mentors and a good understanding of physiology.

Diabetes Supplies

Here in the UK we are incredibly lucky because we have free access to healthcare through our NHS system. The system is not perfect, but it keeps each and every one of us with type 1 diabetes alive, and it provides medical consultations. The NHS is a political pawn and is constantly in the press for the things it does not deliver, and we forget to be grateful for the fantastic services it does provide to us.

The imperfections in the NHS can cause us some difficulties. A couple of common issues that people with type 1 diabetes struggle with in the UK are getting access to insulin pumps and getting enough blood glucose test strips each month, due to cost-saving exercises. Both of these things have been an issue for me in the past and I still see regular posts and media articles for these issues. I decided that I could join the online communities in complaining about what we don't have access to, or I could take some positive action. You have probably already guessed that I decided that positive action was the only viable option, so I volunteered to help INPUT Diabetes (a brilliant charity) which helped me gain access to an insulin pump. I wrote an article for their website, petitioning doctors to prescribe adequate blood glucose test strips; which you can find at www.inputdiabetes.org.uk/glucose-monitoring/access-to-test-strips/ I now regularly attend the Welsh Assembly, taking the concerns of people with type 1 diabetes to the policy makers, who can directly influence how the health service is set up, run, and managed in the country that I live in.

At times when your prescription is not right it can be extremely stressful, but remember getting your prescription fixed is easy. Many doctors these days run a computer system that helps them to manage the task of prescribing medicines and the rules within these computer systems often over ride what we think we need. So the next time your prescription is not what you expect speak to the doctor immediately to make sure that you both understand what you need and why you need it. Remember that, in the UK, there are 400,000 people with type 1 diabetes and just over 40,000 general practitioners. Statistically, each doctor has ten people with type 1 diabetes in his or her case load and over 100 people with type 2 diabetes. We understand that our treatment needs are very different from those with type 2 diabetes, but, with the workload that these doctors have and the number of medical conditions they are expected to be knowledgeable in, it is easy for some of them to see diabetes as a collective community of a single medical condition, rather than separate and distinct conditions. I am not sure how this relates to other parts of the world. However, I do see a lot of online posts from people in the USA, asking if anybody in the online community knows of a local doctor who is great with diabetes, so my assumption is that this is a global issue.

TIP

In western and industrialised societies we are great at complaining about the healthcare that we don't have. It is all too easy to develop an attitude that we are entitled to the gold standard in healthcare. I believe that it is essential that we all have the best health care available to us, but the quality of my healthcare and of my life have improved beyond recognition since I changed my attitude to one where I am humble enough to accept help and be thankful for the care and help I receive. It is still OK for me to seek better health care and improved outcomes but now I do this from an attitude of gratitude.

Managing Your Diabetes Clinic

If you browse through any online discussion group, typically you will see that when people have to attend diabetes clinics there is a feeling of distress. People are publicly stating that they are concerned about the results of their latest HbA1c test (notice that the word test that has appeared here is already associated with negative connotations). I used to have a similar view, but these days my opinion of HbA1c measurements is that they are a fantastic tool for providing me with feedback about how well my lifestyle and strategies have been serving me in the last three months. I cannot get a bad HbA1c result, since what I get is feedback which empowers me to either carry on with my current strategies or to make changes. The journey to this approach requires that we not only make our own shift in perception, but we must also educate our healthcare teams to think in the same way.

For those of us on insulin pumps many of us have faced the threat, either directly or implied, that our pumps will no longer continue to be funded if our HbA1c test results do not demonstrate that the pump is an improvement over multiple daily injections. You must be prepared to demonstrate that your insulin pump is offering you benefits, even if these are not obvious in a standard clinical setting. It is worth keeping records to show why you went onto a pump in the first place, and you should definitely question the authorities on how the decision to change to multiple daily injections will improve your health. You can gently remind the medical team that the first duty of a healthcare professional is to do no harm. Then ask your healthcare team to demonstrate how any change to your diabetes care plan is going to positively impact your health. If they cannot, they have no right to change your treatment plan. Unless removing your access to a pump is going to benefit your health, your medical team is breaking a number of professional codes of conduct if they attempt to do this, and you should remind them of this possible misconduct if they make a threat, no matter how shielded or subtle it is. It's also worth noting that, in the UK, the Secretary of State for Health has endorsed a healthcare policy for those with long-term health issues (such as diabetes) of 'no decision about me, without me', which aims to make patients key stakeholders in their own healthcare.

In the UK we now have a charter that says that you must receive 15 essential diabetes clinical checks each year. The team that put this guidance together have probably never lived a single day with diabetes and have never attended a diabetes clinic as a patient. Like many things, the essential 15 healthcare checks were put together by people with good intentions, and they are promoting early screening for complications, which should be commended. However, they neglect the feelings of the patient. After 37 years of attending hospital appointments I can tell you that being poked, prodded, told that you have gained/lost too much weight, your blood pressure is too high, your cholesterol is too high, your HbA1c is too high, and your lipid levels are too high have lost their novelty and can be filled with negative connotations. Who wants to attend a session like this? As far as I can tell, these 15 checks are used as a box-ticking audit trail, so that the various monitoring systems, the media, and the political entities, including Diabetes UK, can make bold statements about how the system is failing us. I am certain the system does fail us, but, for those with type 1 diabetes, this failure has much more to do with the culture of healthcare than these individual checks.

So how can you get the most from your diabetes consultations? In the first instance, you must recognise that your diabetes care team are not there to judge you; their job is to advise and coach you on achieving the best possible management of your health. If you feel that you are being judged, then you must make your doctor aware of this. Remind him or her that your diabetes is like a sport, in which your diabetes care team are coaches, because they have the expert knowledge and can advise you on how to achieve the best results possible for yourself. Ask your doctor to avoid using language that is suggestive of blame and failure; instead, you want language that empowers you. It is OK to measure my HbA1c and demonstrate that, over the past three months, my diabetes management has not been great, but I don't live life in the past, only in the present and in the future. I need the tools and strategies to help me improve my next result, so how are you going to help me to do that?

Tell your healthcare team that you expect their very best care and attention, and, in exchange for this, you will give them your very best care and attention. Prepare for the consultation like you would any other meeting of highly skilled professional people, even if you have never attended school or worked in your life. You are a highly skilled professional in diabetes, since what other profession demands your attention 24 hours a day, 7 days a week, 365 days a year and does not give you any money or holiday? You are the world's leading expert in your own diabetes; nobody else lives your life or has had your experience of diabetes.

> **TIP**
>
> Remember the words of Elliot P. Joslin *"The person with diabetes who knows about diabetes lives the longest"*. The best gift you can give yourself or your loved one is to become an expert in your own experience of diabetes. The fastest way to do this is to find a great coach or mentor.

When attending the hospital for a consultation you are chairing a meeting with healthcare professionals, who are given the opportunity and privilege to impress you with their ability to look at very personal and intimate information about you. They can make suggestions about how you can improve your health in the long and short term, but it is really all about you. The consultation is your opportunity to talk candidly about the challenges of living with diabetes, and you do not have to meet the expectations of your clinical team, in fact, they must meet your expectations. If you enter your diabetes consultation and you are not treated with the utmost respect,

I suggest that you should sit passively and quietly, offering no input to the meeting. You will eventually be asked what is wrong. This is your opportunity to tell your healthcare team to move away from their desks, computers, and other machines that go 'ping', on which they record statistics about you. After they have moved away, tell them to talk to you with the respect that you deserve. Your healthcare team are being paid for their expert knowledge and to advise you – they are not paid to gather data! You must choose your words carefully and you must show respect in order to earn mutual respect. You should attend the clinic with the mindset that you have hired a team of experts who have opinions about the best way to deal with the challenges that you are facing. Listen to their advice in the spirit that it is intended, and try it out if it is appropriate. If it works – great, if not, discard it. There is no such thing as failure; there are only lessons which teach us that other strategies might serve us better.

I am blessed to be able to get healthcare when I need it, regardless of my ability to pay, and, for this, I am truly grateful for the healthcare service in the UK. In my journey with diabetes my gift is one of an in-depth understanding of my condition and is borne of many years of experience. I now use my own appointments to challenge the boundaries of my self-knowledge and of my healthcare team. I am humble enough to accept that there are things about my own diabetes that I do not know, but every day is an opportunity to learn. Sometimes, there are patterns in my control, which are only obvious to an observer who is not emotionally attached to the results, and this is where the value of my diabetes healthcare conferences really lay for me. My diabetes care team are amazing and they are used to me attending a clinic to discuss ideas of how I can improve my own care or how I can use various strategies to take part in whatever crazy challenge I will undertake next.

> **TIP**
>
> Remember no matter how bad your day has been, no matter what challenges your diabetes has given you today, it has not beaten you. You are a walking miracle. Part of the machinery that is essential to keeping you alive does not function, and you have taken positive steps to manage your diabetes – for that you are awesome. What standards are you willing to accept?

CHAPTER FIVE

NUTRITION

An 87 year old homeless man was interviewed for a TV programme back in the 1970s. In spite of his homeless state and his age, the man was a picture of glowing health, and he told the story of how he asked the market stallholders for the fruit and vegetables that were passed their best at the end of each day. When asked by the interviewer on why he looked so amazing in spite of his age and homeless status, he replied. **'I don't eat junk food; if I don't look after my body, I will have nowhere left to live.'** We can all learn from his amazing philosophy on life and we can aspire to his standards. After all, if a homeless man can make the time and resources to have a healthy diet, what excuse is there for anybody else?

I have been seeing dieticians regularly since I was five years old. In my experience, they provide a useful service in helping people with diabetes to understand the difference between simple and complex carbohydrates, in teaching people to measure, weigh, count and estimate carbohydrates. Unfortunately, as far as I am concerned in relation to diabetes, the service these incredibly talented people provide ends there. The service that I have experienced from dieticians has been far below the standards that I demand for my own health. I believe that dieticians are required to reinforce government and World Health Organisation (WHO) policy on diet; unfortunately, these policies are financially and politically motivated. Let me give you an example: Everybody who has access to newspapers, television, education or the Internet has heard the campaign 'consume five portions of fruit or vegetables a day', but where does this advice really come from? According to the Daily Mail, on 11 January 2011. 'It started as a marketing campaign dreamt up by around 20 fruit and veg companies and the U.S National Cancer Institute at a meeting in California in 1991. And it's been remarkably successful.'

The evidence suggests that five portions of fruit and vegetables per person, per day are woefully inadequate. We see that people who consume much higher levels of vegetables in their diet enjoy better health and typically lead healthier lifestyles. I believe the campaign for five portions of fruit and vegetables a day is good in engaging people to start eating more fruit and vegetables. If you live on a diet of chips and beef burgers and you eat your five a day, it is like smoking 80 cigarettes a day and walking to the shop to buy those cigarettes. The walk is going to give you health benefits, but it won't offer you any real protection from the damage caused by smoking in the first place.

I have improved my nutritional standards to the point where I have an abundance of energy and vitality; I sleep for about five and a half hours a night and I wake up feeling amazing. I don't feel sleepy or tired in the afternoon and the people around me who are not living with a chronic health condition cannot keep up with the hours of work and play that I fit into each day. I am going to provide you with a host of information and resources about nutrition and, depending upon your own standards, you will either dismiss my claims as nonsense or you will investigate my arguments and make your own conclusions, based upon the evidence.

Why do humans believe that they need to consume cow's milk in order to live a healthy life? Why do we believe that milk gives us strong bones? The answer is that we have been indoctrinated to believe this since birth; in fact, this indoctrination began with our parents, grandparents and perhaps even our great grandparents. Milk is even given to school children by education authorities because of its essential health benefits. Which animals in nature consumes the milk of another species? In rare circumstances a maternal animal will adopt the infant of another species and allow it to suckle from them but this is both rare and time limited.

You were born to drink your mother's milk and baby cows were also born to drink their mother's milk – that is the nature of mammals; we suckle our young to the age of weaning. You were born to drink your mother's milk; as an infant it was the perfect food for you. You were 'designed' for it, and it was 'designed' for you. The milk of any other species is perfect for that species and, in exceptional circumstances, might be offered to human infants, but is far from perfect.

You are not supposed to drink milk beyond the age of weaning. It is not natural, and, for most people in the world, they stop secreting an enzyme called lactase into the small intestine somewhere between the ages of two and five years old. This enzyme is essential in enabling us to digest the milk sugar lactose. Have you ever wondered why so many people seem to be lactose intolerant? Lactose intolerance is not a medical condition; it is normal physiology. The ability to produce lactate after weaning requires a genetic mutation on chromosome two.

There is a growing body of evidence that people with type 1 diabetes have an elevated immune response to Bovine

Serum Antibodies (BSA). Bovine Serum Antibodies are found in most dairy products, and, statistically speaking, the evidence that dairy products are one of the triggers which cause type 1 diabetes is extremely significant. The China Study argues that there is an 11 to 13 times greater risk for genetically predisposed children to develop type 1 diabetes if they consume cow's milk. To put this into perspective, if you smoke you only have a ten times greater risk or developing lung cancer than nonsmokers. I accept that Bovine Serum Antibodies theory has a number of flaws, but incidence of type 1 diabetes in countries where dairy is commonly consumed is high (such as Sweden, the USA and the UK) but in countries and regions where dairy is not consumed the incidence of type 1 diabetes is much lower. Is this a coincidence?

I cannot tell you that milk is the trigger for type 1 diabetes or that it does not have any impact, but I can encourage you to read the studies for yourself and remain open-minded. However, let's be conservative here: There is a risk that milk might trigger type 1 diabetes, but there is no risk associated with avoiding dairy. You must choose for yourself: I have made my assessment, I refuse to eat or drink foods containing dairy and I encourage my family to do the same. If you already have type 1 diabetes new evidence suggests that you may still retain some islets of Langerhans cells which produce insulin. Therefore, if dairy is a trigger for type 1 diabetes, could avoiding dairy help you preserve some of this cell line and its function? In case you find the concept that there may be a link between type 1 and cow's milk difficult to accept just enter the following search into Google 'cow's milk type 1 diabetes' and read the articles for and against the theory. There is enough doubt in my mind to mark dairy food as high risk.

How will I get calcium if I don't consume dairy? Calcium is essential for all humans, because it is an ionic salt used in electrical signal conduction throughout the body; in fact, the chances are that if you ever had a cramp in a muscle, it is because you were deficient in calcium. The biggest stores of calcium in your body are your bones and, in times of calcium deficit, the calcium reservoirs in your bones will be used to supplement the available calcium. The China Study demonstrated that countries which consume the highest amount of dairy have the highest incidence of osteoporosis, and in countries and regions where milk is not consumed, osteoporosis is a rare condition. This is interesting when you consider that people with type 1 diabetes have an elevated lifetime risk of osteoporosis. Could we mitigate this by avoiding dairy even though this seems counterintuitive?

The good news is that calcium is readily available in green vegetables, particularly spinach and kale. The even better news is that a diet rich in green, live plant based foods provides us with plenty of calcium, and it is instrumental in reversing coronary heart disease, according to the work and research of Dr Dean Ornish. In his work with patients with severe cardiovascular disease, Dr Ornish was able to manage and even reverse the narrowing of the arteries which supply the heart with oxygenated blood using diet alone. It is the narrowing of these arteries that causes thousands of heart attacks and thousands of patients to go through cardiac bypass surgery. Therefore, as a person with diabetes, I prefer to consume my calcium by consuming green vegetables. This means that I get plenty of calcium, and I may be offered some protection from vascular disease, which is a secondary symptom of diabetes. In addition to this I am not filling my body with a lot of saturated animal fats found in dairy products, which would significantly increase my risk of cardiovascular disease.

TIP

Coeliac disease is seen in about 1% of the population, but about 10% of all people with type 1 diabetes have Coeliac disease. If you have type 1 diabetes, and you have not already been tested, please get a simple blood test performed by your doctor to include or exclude Coeliac disease. You may have Coeliac disease without even knowing it, but the constant inflammatory immune response is going to make managing your blood glucose levels impossible. Untreated Coeliac disease can cause a huge variety of serious symptoms, including infertility and even cancer of the gut. Treatment is simple and pain free, since you just need to avoid gluten and foods containing gluten.

I appreciate that everybody with diabetes has always been led down a path of eating a diet which is based primarily on complex carbohydrates. If you stop and think about this for just a moment does it actually make any sense?

You need insulin to perform normal metabolic functions in the body, which are largely related to ensuring that there is always enough energy to maintain function of the nervous system and reproductive system. However, much of the insulin that we take is used to metabolise carbohydrates. But before anybody complains, I fully acknowledge that insulin is used to metabolise proteins and fats. Nevertheless, the more we load the body with carbohydrates, the more insulin we need, and the more insulin we take, the more variability we see in its actions. The only way we can predict, with any certainty, what the insulin is going to do is to reduce the amount we take. I have been using an insulin pump for seven years and I am an advocate of promoting the use of insulin pumps. I have been trained in DAFNE (Dose Adjustment For Normal Eating) and it is true that you can compensate for high carbohydrate diets with large doses of insulin, but it has been my experience that I cannot do this without having huge variability in blood glucose levels. I have observed this same variability in blood glucose levels in other people with diabetes, who comment that they have very high or very low blood glucose levels on a regular basis.

I have tried a whole variety of nutrition strategies to maintain the best blood glucose levels with the least transients, and for me, the best have been low carbohydrate regimes. Let me make this absolutely clear, I am not talking about the Atkins diet, I am not even talking about the diet suggested by Dr Richard Bernstein, though I would recommend that everybody with type 1 diabetes should read Dr Bernstein's book. Particularly, you should read his section on the rule of small numbers, which can be summarised as 'big inputs make big mistakes, small inputs make small mistakes.' Bernstein argues that large portions of carbohydrates lead to large doses of insulin and variability on measuring carbohydrate quantities, and to variability on insulin action. The accuracy of blood glucose measurements becomes very significant when those numbers are high, but are much less significant when

TYPE 1 DIABETES And How To Live With It

those numbers are small. Whilst I did not find his nutritional approach acceptable for me because of the high volume of animal protein, I did and I do follow his principles of a low carbohydrate diet most of the time.

> ## TIP
>
> Try a nutritional approach that is low in carbohydrates and high in live plant based foods and your insulin requirements will be amazingly low, and your energy levels amazingly high. However, before making changes like this, unless you are competent and proficient at adjusting your insulin requirements, get support from your healthcare team in managing your diabetes. Some diabetes specialists disregard the work of Dr Bernstein, but in his defence, he was diagnosed with type 1 diabetes in 1946 and still works as an endocrinologist today; how many of your healthcare team have lived with type 1 diabetes for 70 years? Did I forget to mention that he claims to have reversed many of the complications of diabetes he was suffering from back in the early 1970s, including retinopathy?

My own strategy is based on the requirements of human nutrition. This means that I consume foods that in evolutionary terms have been the staples of the human diet, and I eat seasonally. Whilst I cannot get the exact crops and meats of earlier times I can simulate many of them. I can ensure that my diet is free from dairy; has minimal carbohydrates; contains whole live plants, such as spinach, kale and broccoli. If I cook vegetables, I cook them for only a minimal amount of time. Everybody should try 'frightened broccoli', which involves steaming broccoli over boiling water for a couple of minutes and then drizzling some olive oil and a sprinkling of salt – it is absolutely delicious. Even my 11 year old daughter, who believes that vegetables are a form of poison, loves frightened broccoli. I avoid foods which were not part of the evolutionary chain, such as white potatoes and wheat. This conveniently provides me with the most amazingly nourishing diet, without the need to consume carbohydrates like they are going out of fashion.

I am not vegetarian, though I did live with a vegan diet for 18 months. I do eat high quality meats and free range eggs, but I certainly don't consume them everyday. I minimise the amount of fruit that I eat because of the high carbohydrate content. I have been working with Eric Edmeades and he has coached me to a nutritional approach where my blood glucose levels are incredibly stable, my insulin requirements are amazingly small and my energy levels have soared to levels that I never thought were possible. In addition to all of this my HbA1c levels have dropped by 15%; my blood pressure has dropped by 20 points and my cholesterol levels, which were always low anyway, have dropped. You might be forgiven for thinking that you cannot consume a low carbohydrate diet and perform a strenuous or physical activity without going hypo, but I was already consuming a low carbohydrate diet when I ran my first half marathon, and I maintained extremely stable blood glucose levels throughout.

There have only been two occasions in my life when my blood glucose levels have been consistently well maintained, and on both occasions, I have followed a low carbohydrate diet, once by following Dr Bernstein's low carb, high protein diet, and the other time, by following the Eric Edmeades programme. I found that Bernstein's diet was difficult to comply with and I was eating more animal protein than I could tolerate. However, Eric's programme provides a lot of live plant based food and products and some animal proteins (these are optional but recommended) There are many fantastic nutrition programmes out there, and some even claim that they can cure type 2 diabetes. The Raw for Thirty Days programme, which I have never followed, even claims to have 'cured' both type 1 and 2 diabetes. We have seen multiple examples of people becoming asymptomatic for type 2 diabetes, but the evidence is less clear for type 1; in fact, when looking at the Raw for Thirty Days programme, I could not determine if the patients using insulin were people with type 2 diabetes who need to use insulin or, in fact, had type 1 diabetes.

In summary, if you want to manage your diabetes effectively you need to look very closely at your diet and how the things you are eating today affect your blood glucose levels in the hours and days ahead. I understand that this is a controversial chapter, but please try to have an open mind and try a low carbohydrate diet. In a non diabetic person insulin is mostly produced according to the amount of fuel that is consumed. Why should you be any different? Why do you load up your body with masses of insulin, and then try to eat the correct amount of carbohydrates, so that they are absorbed at the right time to match the peak of the insulin action profile? This is not a natural way to eat or take insulin, and yet people with diabetes and their healthcare professionals are always surprised when this strategy does not work. You are metabolically disadvantaged in respect to consuming large amounts of carbohydrates, please stop punishing your body by pretending that you can eat normally, even if you are using an insulin pump. It is true that I can eat the occasional high carbohydrate meal, and I can get away with it for a day or two, but when I try to do this consistently my diabetes management becomes a Herculean task.

CHAPTER SIX

EXERCISE

Diabetes and exercise are always difficult partners. We are told that we must exercise to maintain cardiovascular health, a healthy weight, insulin sensitivity and to keep cholesterol levels in target. However, as you start an exercise programme, you usually find that you have an increased number of hypos, and if you are anything like me, a huge increase in the incidence and severity of night time hypoglycaemia. It can often feel like exercise is counterintuitive in insulin dependant diabetes, because you cannot possibly lose weight if, for every calorie that you burn in exercise, you need to eat a bar of chocolate to treat or prevent a hypo. When you wake up a day or two after an exercise session with that morning-after-the-night-before feeling (when you did not have the benefit of the night before) which you get when you have slept through a hypo, and your head feels foggy, your body feels heavy, and the effort of walking from the bedroom to the bathroom is more difficult than running ten miles, you really start to question if this exercising business is good for your health. It certainly doesn't appear to be any help in managing glucose levels.

How can you move from these feelings of isolation and despair around exercise? Especially as many of us don't particularly enjoy the idea of exercise and diabetes offers us a convenient opt-out clause for any exercise session? How can you move to a situation where you enjoy exercise and use it as part of your strategy for managing your diabetes? Each sport places different demands upon us and the intensity and type of exercise will change the way in which you need to think about preparing for exercise, participating in exercise, and managing the hours and even days after an exercise session. We all need to find a form of exercise that we love: It might be walking the dog, playing in the park, or rowing in the Olympics. It does not matter what exercise you do, just that you do some, as one of my nutrition coaches once said to me. 'The difference between the living and the dead is that dead people don't move!'

My preferred forms of exercise include hillwalking and running half marathons. Many of you will be looking at this thinking that there is no way that you could run a half marathon or walk up three mountains consecutively. You are, of course, absolutely right; you cannot do it for two reasons: (1) you have decided that you cannot, and (2) you have not trained, planned and prepared to do it. Your diabetes may seem like a barrier to exercise, and I used to think this way too, but I started to ask different questions about exercise and I identified people with diabetes who were performing exceptionally in their chosen sport.

Initially during my hillwalking my blood glucose levels would drop and stopping to recover was tedious and it slowed the whole group down. This is not a big problem in good weather, but when it is freezing cold or raining, standing on a hillside for 20 minutes waiting for blood glucose levels to raise can become dangerous. So what changed? I looked for an athlete who has diabetes, uses insulin, and performs at the highest level, and I asked how can they do these things? The first person I identified was Sir Steven Redgrave and I visited his website, remembering that success always leaves clues. I quickly found links to the diabetes specialist team that helped Sir Steven with his diabetes in his rowing career and they have a fantastic website. I spent hours reading all of the different cases that were on the website looking for a common theme, and I began to try to emulate the strategies that people were telling me. I enjoyed considerable success in this, but I was still having hypos, and they would continue sporadically for a few days after a long walking session. My improvement in control whilst exercising was good, but far below the standard that I expected.

I emailed the team at www.runsweet.com directly and they were happy to help me. The great news is that for most people living in the UK you can get a referral to this team through the NHS! The level of knowledge that this team has and the strategies they worked out for me were outstanding, and I was able to utilise them. Within just a few months, I had completed the Welsh Three Peaks Challenge, walking Snowdon, Cadair Idris and Pen-Y-Fan in less than 16 hours including the travel, and I did this without any hypos! Whilst hillwalking my strategy looks something like the following:

- Check blood glucose levels before setting out on the walk. If my blood glucose is above 13.1, I give a correction of insulin and wait for the blood glucose to drop to below 13.1. If a correction is needed, be very conservative because a large shot of insulin has a longer action cycle than a small shot of insulin and I really don't want to go hypo two hours into a walk up a mountain.

- Once my blood glucose is in target, I reduce my basal insulin to 20 percent half an hour before I start walking.

Sorry guys, if you are using multiple daily injections, you can't do this bit, unless you plan the night before!

- I wear a heart rate monitor whilst walking and limit my pace to a maximum of 80 percent of cardiovascular maximum rate. Your cardiovascular maximum rate is 220 beats per minute minus your age. If you are 25 years old, this means 220 beats per minute – 25 years = 195 beats per minute. If you are 40 years old, it means 220 beats per minute – 40 years = 180 beats per minute. So taking the example of a 40-year-old, the maximum pace would be 220 beats per minute – 40 years = 180 beats per minute, but our target is actually 80 percent of cardiovascular maximum, so we then get 180 x 80 percent = 144 beats per minute.

- Set a timer alarm and stop every 30 minutes to perform a blood glucose measurement. This is important because it shows the trend that your blood glucose level is heading in even without using a continuous glucose monitor. It is essential to write down this result and if blood glucose levels are falling you can with experience predict when a hypo is likely to occur and treat it before it happens. If you are using a continuous glucose monitor make sure it is functioning correctly and is calibrated, and that the readings are consistent with your expectations. It is worth noting that continuous glucose monitors are fantastic, but they only demonstrate trends. A rapidly falling blood glucose may not be demonstrated until you are already experiencing a hypo.

Hillwalking itself presents a challenge in terms of managing blood glucose levels, but to walk three mountains consecutively when on the Welsh three peaks was particularly challenging for blood glucose levels. There is never enough time between each of the peaks to recover the glycogen levels in the liver and muscle cells before the next mountain. As the challenge progresses, preventing hypos becomes progressively harder, although I managed to complete the challenge in 15 hours without a single hypo. My plan for doing this involved several strategies: (1) massive loading of complex carbohydrates the day before the event, (2) running my basal insulin at an 80 percent reduction whilst ascending the hills, (3) taking blood glucose measurements every 30 minutes during the event, and (4) treating falling blood glucose levels before hypos occurred. During the descent from the mountains my basal rates were returned to normal levels and large meals loaded with complex carbohydrates were consumed whilst travelling from one mountain to the next. After finishing the event, my basal insulin levels were reduced to 60 percent on the first and second days and to 80 percent on the third day.

I am extremely lucky and grateful that I have an insulin pump, it gives me the ability to make precise and relatively quick-acting adjustments to my insulin delivery to help me participate in sports. It would still be possible to participate in my chosen sports if I was using daily injections, but I would need to plan my strategies for exercise at least 12 hours in advance to make changes to my long-acting insulin. As a pump user I don't have any long-acting insulin, more on this in the next chapter.

In exercise terms there are three main heart rate zones: The fat burning zone, the aerobic zone and the anaerobic zone. To work them out precisely you need a physiology laboratory that can measure the gasses that you breathe in and out whilst your heart rate is measured as you exercise. Since most of us don't have access to this kind of equipment we can use a heart rate monitor and some calculations, which give us general indications of the ranges. Heart rate monitors usually consist of a chest strap that has a transmitter on it and a watch that receives the signals from the chest strap. You can avoid this level of expense by carefully observing yourself. Whilst exercising if you can hold a normal conversation, you are typically in your fat burning zone; if you can hold a conversation, but the sentences have pauses between them and are typically quite short, you are in your aerobic zone; if holding a conversation is impossible, you are in your anaerobic zone. I have learned through my own challenges and running that working within the aerobic heart rate zone is essential.

TIP

A heart rate monitor is essential to successfully managing your diabetes whilst you exercise. As your heart rate changes, the rate at which you burn sugar also changes, and the type of sugar you burn is also dependent upon your heart rate. Basic heart rate monitors are relatively cheap and that is all that you need.

When I work in the anaerobic zones I inevitably find that my blood glucose levels drop rapidly and hypos are then a problem for me. This does not mean that I cannot work in the anaerobic zones; it simply means that I need to limit the amount of time that I work in those zones.

When you are exercising in an aerobic capacity you need to consume between 30 and 60 grams of carbohydrate per hour to maintain blood glucose levels. When I walk in the hills I find that dried mango is amazing for doing this: It tastes good, is really high in fructose (fruit sugar), is light weight and travels well. Unfortunately when I run I just cannot chew and swallow dried food, so I rely on sports drinks. Commercially available brands in the supermarkets, such as Gatorade and Lucozade Sport, are not well suited to this because they only contain about six percent glucose. Therefore, to consume 60 grams of carbohydrates an hour, I would need to drink a litre per hour. The issues here are that I cannot carry that much when running for two or three hours and I cannot drink that much. Consuming 60 grams of carbohydrate an hour is the upper limit of how much glucose the body can absorb and can often leave you feeling nauseous. The solution is to use a sports drink made for the cycling community, which contains much higher glucose concentrations; these drinks have been formulated to contain not only glucose but a variety of ionic salts (electrolytes), which promote absorption of glucose. Glucose gels can work well, but some people find them difficult to digest.

> **TIP**
>
> A glucose transmitter substance, called, GLUT 4, is released during exercise. GLUT 4 allows a muscle cell to transfer glucose across the cell membrane without requiring insulin; in effect, you are more

sensitive to insulin. It is also worth noting that muscles contain a store of glycogen that appears to act as an immediate store of energy for the muscles, which they release when the muscles is called upon to do work. After you have exercise, these glycogen stores are depleted, and the muscles will replenish them. It has so far been my experience that this appears to happen in the early hours of the morning for each of the next two nights. This can cause nighttime hypoglycaemia, and, after a long endurance walk or run, I reduce by basal insulin overnight; for those using multiple daily injections, this is your long acting insulin. I believe that different forms of exercise like weight lifting or sprinting would change the timing of this glycogen replenishment to the pre-dawn hours.

If you are struggling to deal with diabetes and exercise you will find some excellent advice available from your diabetes specialist healthcare team. There is a wealth of experience in the online forums of people who are living with diabetes and performing at outstanding levels in sports.

There are fantastic books and websites on exercise and diabetes, and, like everything else related to diabetes, there are no simple and easy answers. We must all find our own path based upon our own fitness and the type of exercise that we do and the duration of that exercise. However the general principles are well understood. Dr Ian Gallen is a world-leading expert on diabetes and exercise and I would recommend that you visit his website www.runsweet.com as a starting point for information. My own journey with exercise has been an on/off affair at various times in my life and it is really only in the last five years that I have decided to empower myself to perform in endurance events. This has taken me on a journey of reading medical physiology, understanding the requirement for insulin in exercise, and understanding how heart rate affects the type and rate at which we burn fuels, e.g., glucose burning, fat burning, aerobic respiration and anaerobic respiration.

Understanding a little of the basic science of exercise will help you to appreciate why exercise gives you such a challenge if you have type 1 diabetes. Your body prefers to use glucose as its energy source; it is for this reason that people are advised to carbohydrate load before an endurance event. However, your body only has about five grams of glucose available to it at any one time and this gets burned pretty quickly. When the glucose is burned, blood glucose levels start to drop and glucagon release from the pancreas occurs (even in people with diabetes), which then releases glycogen from the liver and the muscles. The glycogen in the muscles only acts locally to fuel the muscles, but the glycogen from the liver has a massive cascade effect and it raises the blood glucose levels substantially.

It seems counterintuitive, but if you don't have enough insulin on board before you start to exercise, your blood glucose levels can actually increase as a result of exercise and could even put you at risk of going into Diabetic Ketoacidosis (DKA). This process is called glycogenolysis, and it is promoted by the feedback relationship between insulin and glucagon from the pancreas, but adrenaline (epinephrine) will also promote glycogenolysis as part of the flight or fight response, resulting in an increased blood glucose level that gives the body the fuel it needs to perform. The challenge is that as a person with diabetes you must be sure that you have enough insulin on board to deal with this process without having so much insulin that you will go hypo.

TIP

The science part here is a very simplified explanation of the actual physiology but it is still complex. You don't need to understand and remember it all. The key point is to make sure that you have enough insulin available when you start exercising so that your body can utilize the fuels properly. The challenge is that exercise will make you much more sensitive to insulin so you need to be more conservative at treating high blood glucose levels when you are planning to exercise. Normal protocols suggest that you should never start to exercise if your blood glucose levels are over 13.1 mmols/L because there is a risk that you could develop Ketoacidosis. This occurs because there is already an insulin deficit and when you start exercising glucose supplies are released from the muscles and the liver – and if your blood glucose levels are too high this can make matters worse.

Don't forget that exercise is not necessarily running a half marathon. Doing the housework, walking to the park, playing on the swings or trampoline, running for the bus and a million other tasks are all forms of exercise. Children typically take part in more exercise than adults; often it is for short durations as they run up the road, or play in the park, or even jump up and down on the bed. Next time you wonder why that hypo occurred, don't forget all of those simple daily activities that made you move and changed your heart rate.

CHAPTER SEVEN

MANAGING DIABETES

In this chapter I will take you through my own journey of treatment and I will discuss the pros and cons as I have found them. I cannot give you a prescription for how you should take your own insulin because I am not a medical doctor. Before we start getting too involved in this discussion, we need to get a few definitions out of the way.

Term	Definition
Animal insulin	Insulin derived typically from cows (bovine insulin) or from pigs (porcine insulin) for use in humans.
Human insulin	Genetically manufactured human insulin for clinical use.
Analogue insulin	Insulin based upon human insulin that has been genetically engineered by changing the protein structure, which changes its action profile.
MDI	Multiple Daily Injections, usually 4 or more injections a day, often using a pen-like device.

Insulin pump	A small mechanical device connected to you 24 hours a day, which delivers insulin to a pre-programmed pattern.
Bolus	A dose of short-acting insulin given with a meal or to treat a high blood glucose level.
Basal	A dose of insulin for basal metabolic requirements; for those on MDI, it is a long-acting insulin given once or twice each day; for those on an insulin pump, it is rapidly acting insulin that is constantly delivered in small quantities by the pump.

Most people starting their journey with type 1 diabetes begin with daily insulin injections. These days it seems quite common for people, even young children, to have multiple insulin injections each day. This is call MDI therapy (Multiple Daily Injections) You might ask, 'Why so many injections?' 'Why can't we have just one injection?' You will, of course, remember from our earlier discussion that insulin is a protein and cannot be taken orally because it would get digested by the stomach before it becomes active.

In 1977 I used to have just one injection each day of an insulin called Monotard. It was a long-acting insulin and, at the time of my own diagnosis, human insulin was not yet available. I had to be injected with bovine (cow) insulin, which kept me alive, but it gave me huge hives at the injection sites. When I reflect upon this I often wonder if this is related to the hypothesis that bovine serum antibodies may be the trigger for type 1 diabetes and I may have had an immune response to something in the bovine insulin – of course, it may have just been the poor purification processes, stabilisers, and preservatives that where in use back then. I was quickly swapped to porcine insulin and my allergic reaction was far less severe. I remained on a single injection per day for seven years, so why don't we do this anymore?

The insulin that I was taking was a long-acting insulin by the standards of the day. However we know that even the modern analogue long-acting insulins, such as Levemir and Lantus, cannot give us insulin that has an action profile covering us for 24 hours a day. Research suggests that in the best cases we can get coverage for about 20 hours; therefore, a single injection a day gives us at least four hours in each day where there is no active insulin. There is another problem with this treatment protocol. Giving a long-acting insulin only provides a background level of insulin but each time food is consumed, there will be huge climbs in blood glucose levels. Measuring blood glucose levels two hours after a meal is called a postprandial test and is now seen as an important indication of how well your insulin therapy is matched to your diet. Postprandial blood glucose measurements are also seen as important contributions to your long-term blood glucose measurements in the HbA1c measurement. To combat the problem of high postprandial glucose levels you would need such high doses of a single long-acting insulin that, if you stopped eating for only a few hours, you would have a hypo. Welcome to the world I grew up in, eating small meals six times a day and having any one of these meals just 30 minutes late would lead to severe hypoglycaemia.

Genetically manufactured human insulin became available in the UK in the early 1980s and I was an early adopter. The change was remarkably positive for me, and yet, to this day I see articles being posted by people who want to return to animal-based insulin products because they have less hypo awareness on human and analogue insulins. For me I will probably never go back to animal insulin since the hives, itching and completely unpredictable nature of absorption are things that I never want to experience again. I can only speak from my own experiences and perspective, but I wonder if those who return to animal insulin for hypo awareness reasons are getting improved awareness as a result of the insulin or as a result of their blood glucose levels running slightly higher due to slower or impaired insulin absorption. We know that the more hypo episodes a person experiences, the less hypo awareness they have and this can be recovered relatively quickly by avoiding hypos for a few months, e.g., a clinically managed short-term episode of running higher blood glucose levels.

As a young child I would frequently end up in hospital with Diabetic Ketoacidosis (DKA) as a result of the poor control offered to me by the single shot of long-acting insulin and the fact that home blood glucose monitoring did not exist. During one of these episodes, when I was about 11 years old, I asked if I could go onto two injections a day to improve my control. I then began using Actrapid insulin, a short-acting insulin, and Monotard. Suddenly my injections were more complex, as I had to draw insulin from both vials into a single syringe. This meant that I had to be really careful not to contaminate the short-acting insulin with the long-acting insulin and vice versa. Getting the air out of the syringe without losing insulin was a skill I mastered quickly, because if insulin was lost how would I know if it was short-acting or long-acting insulin? This change to two injections each day made a huge difference to my life. I could suddenly move a meal by 30 minutes and not collapse with a hypo because I could delay my injection a little. When I was on a single injection each day we had to make sure that each day my insulin shot was given by 07:00 a.m., regardless of whether it was Saturday, Sunday, or even Christmas Day. Now for the first time I could actually sleep until 07:30 in the morning. I soon realised that the extra burden of another injection each day had given me some freedom. I could sleep later, I could eat later, and I could even adjust my insulin a little if I was eating more carbohydrates.

I continued on this treatment protocol until I was sixteen and I left school. I had been eager to go to the all new regime of using multiple daily injections by a Novopen for about 18 months, but my clinic refused to allow me to carry insulin at school. So when I left school I immediately went to four injections each day. By now I was so used to injections I could do them in my sleep, and in fact, they were so mundane that I could not tell you if I had done an injection or not. However, the freedom was remarkable, because I could give a shot of short-acting insulin before each meal with a shot of a long-acting insulin before bed. Like all good patients I learned how to use the system diligently, and like all teenagers, I quickly realised that I could abuse this system and really push the limits of what it could do.

I stopped attending diabetes clinic because it was boring. I saw a different doctor each time, who knew nothing about me, and, as far as I could tell, even less about diabetes; besides I could get my prescription filled by my family doctor. It was years before I attended diabetes clinic again. At the time I told everybody that I was an expert and I did not need help from a clinic. Whilst at work one day I collapsed with a hypo so severe that I literally passed out. One of my colleagues had been briefed on how best to help me in the event of a hypo and he managed to get me to drink some Coke and bring me round. I had been a burden to all those around me for a while, being complacent about my diabetes, having severe hypos, and passing out on any number of occasions. But it was never once alcohol related! Yet this hypo at work was new territory for me since I was sent home, and over the following days, spent more time passed out than conscious. I stopped taking insulin and still the hypos carried on. I needed help. I had to accept that I was not the expert and so I phoned the hospital.

My Diabetes Specialist Nurse, Jan, had been working with me since I was five, in her usual amazing manner, took everything in her stride. After four days with no insulin I was still passing out with hypoglycaemia, eating anything and everything available, Jan and I developed two theories. The unlikely one was that I was producing insulin again either due to the recovery of islets cells in the pancreas or a tumour. The more likely theory was that my diabetes management was so poor and my doses of long-acting insulin were simply so large that even after four days without a shot I still had masses of insulin in my system.

How is that possible? The larger the dose of insulin that we give the longer its action profile. At that time I had been using a long-acting insulin called Ultratard for my basal insulin shots. My clinic had stopped prescribing it four years previously, because they saw huge numbers of patients collapsing with sustained hypoglycaemia. I had been the victim of my own complacency; if I had attended clinic I would have stopped using this insulin years ago too. My insulin was swapped to a different long-acting product called Insulatard. I would love to say that my diabetes complacency ended then, but it did not.

After this crisis I was careful for a few months, and once again, I began to push the boundaries and rebel against my diabetes. Looking back I can now see that like most people in their late teens and early twenties I was struggling to accept my diabetes, and I wanted to be like everybody else. I was getting judged at home about not going to clinic, and whilst I realised that this was for my own benefit, I did not want to hear it. I failed to learn the lessons that my diabetes, and the universe, was trying to teach me at the time and I carried on regardless. The only difference now was that I conceded to attending clinic (under protest) a couple of times each year. Things carried on this way with having multiple daily injections, eating whatever I liked whenever I liked and exercising without paying any regard to my diabetes. By now I was doing karate, rock climbing, and going to the gym; if I was not working or studying, I was working out. I was tired of going hypo because it made me feel so crappy, and I never wanted to be hypo whilst in the dojo or on the rock face, so I used to run my blood glucose levels high to prevent hypos.

At this time home blood glucose monitoring was available to me. However, I would go for periods where I was fastidious about my diabetes management to periods of rejection and denial, where I did not test my blood glucose levels for weeks or even months on end. I would claim that I knew if my sugars where high or low, because I could feel it. I have news for everybody out there – this is complete and utter crap! It is true that you can feel when your blood glucose levels are different, but if you get used to low blood glucose levels, this becomes normal for you, and if you normally have high blood glucose levels, this becomes your normal. I remember a lot of occasions where I did not believe my test results, because I felt low and my results showed a high reading. Those high readings were in fact low endings for me at the time, because I had set a new internal baseline of very high blood glucose levels and did not even realise it.

My next diabetes crisis was looming, my girlfriend, Denise, had just gone to university and I now had loads of free evenings and weekends. Whilst my diabetes was still wildly out of control I would insist I had great control and, to show this, I was working out in the gym, going swimming, rock climbing, and doing karate. In fact, I was exercising every single day, often a few times each day. I was getting really fit. Then I got a cold, nothing remarkable, so I carried on with my normal complacency, going to work, but cutting back on exercise for a few days. Then one morning I woke up to this feeling that I had somebody sitting on my chest, and with each inspiration of breath, it felt like a knife was being driven through my chest. Breathing had become so painful I could hardly move and so I staggered to the bathroom and got in a hot shower; the moisture in the air seemed to revive me and so I dressed and went to work.

Later that morning I realised it had been a mistake to go to work and I phoned my doctor for an emergency appointment. I was given an examination and sent for chest X-rays. The radiographer told me to go straight back to my doctor, who diagnosed me with pneumonia and pleurisy. My doctor insisted that I needed to be admitted to hospital and made arrangements for an ambulance to take me from surgery into hospital. In my usual complacent fashion, I said, 'Don't worry,

I will make my own arrangements'. I went home with a pack of antibiotics and stayed there, never making that journey to the hospital because I did not want advice and coaching about my diabetes. It was six months before I recovered my fitness and a year before I felt well again.

I had made a remarkable journey, and yet my complacency and lack of acceptance about my diabetes was still controlling all of my actions. I was not managing my diabetes – it was controlling me. A few years later when Denise finished university we moved in together and this was an opportunity for a fresh start, a new doctor, and a referral to a new diabetes care team. By now I had a job which was regularly taking me all over the world. We were travelling a lot for our holidays and we were just about to get married. I attended diabetes clinic for the first time in years, and my new consultant was brilliant. After my HbA1c was measured at 17.1, my diabetes management improved massively and I suddenly understood that my complacency about diabetes was going to kill me. Within 6 months, I had lowered my HbA1c to 8.0 just by changing my attitude towards my diabetes and my blood glucose measurements were looking good. I was still taking multiple daily injections, but, in all honesty, there would be times when I would do a shot and put my syringes away and think – did I just do that shot? I would then look around the site where I thought I might have injected to see if there were any needle marks, or bleeding, or if there was any insulin coming from the injection site. On more occasions than I care to admit, I have not done an injection for fear of doubling my insulin dose, and, on a few occasions, I have done two injections instead of one and suffered the inevitable hypo.

TIP

Even if you are the expert in your own diabetes, always remain humble enough to seek and accept help. You sometimes find help in the most unexpected and unusual places. I have always found that helping other people with their diabetes journeys reinforces my own learning and experiences, and this is one of the reasons I love to help others with diabetes.

Denise and I had been married for three years when we decided to start a family. At the time she was teaching at a primary school and I was travelling the world as an IT consultant. The arrival of our first daughter, Kyla, was a life-changing experience. I had already been diagnosed with background retinopathy and I know the risks associated with long-term type 1 diabetes and loss of eyesight due to retinopathy. As I held my newborn daughter in my arms I decided that I was going to do everything in my power to make sure that I would see my daughter grow up. In that moment my destiny in life was shaped, I already had a lot of knowledge about diabetes, but now I was going to be a world-class expert in my own diabetes.

For the next few years I continued with multiple daily injections, but I had already learned that the gold standard for insulin therapy was an insulin pump and I began to investigate. To begin with my view was that I didn't want something attached to me 24 hours a day, 7 days a week, because insulin pumps are for people who can't manage their diabetes. How do you go to sleep or go swimming, and how do you deal with a hard plastic box that is attached to you with two feet of thin plastic tubing in those intimate moments? To answer the question briefly, sometimes I disconnect it, and other times, there are three of us in the bed (me, Denise, and my pump) with my wife's consent of course. Once again diabetes is giving me an extraordinary life!

I quickly learned that there is a very active and informative blog site for insulin pump users and, if you can think of a question, you can guarantee that somebody on there has an answer. The site is a remarkable source of diabetes knowledge. Without them and Gaynor, my diabetes specialist nurse and an insulin pump user herself, and Vanessa, my dietician who is pump trained, I may not have made the transition to a pump. The blog site is becoming less active these days and I believe this is due to all of the social media on Facebook and Twitter, but I still check the blogs daily and post questions and answers when I can. The website location is www.insulin-pumpers.org.uk, and even if you are not on an insulin pump please join the discussion here. Just about everybody on the site has many years of living with diabetes, both on and off an insulin pump, and the wealth of knowledge and experience is humbling.

Insulin is given in a direct relationship to your body mass (weight), to how active you are, to how many grams of carbohydrates you consume on average each day and to your age. For women their menstrual cycle and whether or not they are pregnant or planning on becoming pregnant will also have an impact, but these events are beyond my experience of diabetes. The general rules of thumb are well understood and can be adapted into excel spreadsheets quickly and easily, so that you can work out what your insulin dose starting point is. You can use these starting points with your historical data of your blood glucose levels and carbohydrate content to make judgements about what modifications you will need to make.

I recommend that you read the book Pumping Insulin by Roberts and Walsh. The last time I checked it cost about £20 on Amazon. You can download it on an e-reader but I find the paper copy is best because the tables and graphs make more sense that way. This book is brilliant if you are on an insulin pump or thinking about getting one. Even if you are not even vaguely interested in a pump, the information here on insulin injections makes this book required reading for anybody living with diabetes.

Insulin pumps are incredible devices in a small package and most of them have some tubing that attaches the pump to a cannula, which is inserted into your skin. The cannula stays inside you for about three days before you need to replace it. The pump contains only short-acting insulin and you programme it to trickle feed small amounts of insulin into you throughout the day and night, to provide you with background or basal insulin. This offers several advantages over long-acting insulin given on MDI: (1) the insulin action covers a full 24 hours, (2) the pump can be programmed to deliver different amounts of insulin at different times of the day to reflect the differing requirements that the body has, but long-acting insulin provides a flat profile throughout the day and night, and cannot accommodate dawn phenomenon, (3) the delivery of background insulin can be adjusted quickly to accommodate exercise or illness. In addition to the delivery of background insulin throughout the day and night, the pump is also used to deliver bolus insulin to deal with meals and high blood glucose levels.

The real advantage here is not that you no longer have to inject, but once the pump is set up with your personal parameters you can enter your blood glucose measurements and the number of carbohydrates that you are about to eat, and the pump will calculate the amount of insulin that you need. It will also discount the amount of insulin that you already have on board, helping to prevent hypoglycaemia. The result is that your blood glucose levels are greatly improved, and although clinically you will probably experience more hypos, they will typically be much less severe. If this does not sell you on an insulin pump the amount of freedom these devices give you over your diabetes is amazing. Whilst my diabetes still responds best to routine, if I decide to miss a meal or eat extra or even fast for a whole day, I can. The downside of using an insulin pump is that the device is connected to you 24 hours a day, 7 days a week, 52 weeks each year. Using an insulin pump requires much higher levels of patient compliance than multiple daily injections do. The need to test blood glucose levels is greater because you have no background insulin. Failure of the pump can and does occur and you need to be able to recognise it and act quickly. I have now been using an insulin pump for seven years and there is no way that I will go back to using multiple daily injections.

In the UK the National Health Service will provide insulin pumps, but there are strict criteria that you must fit before you can be considered for a pump, and you must be supported by your diabetes consultant. Insulin pumps are expensive for the health service to purchase and run and we have only limited evidence to demonstrate that people on insulin pumps have fewer and less severe complications than those not on multiple daily injections. This lack of evidence is because the uptake of insulin pumps is quite low, and they remain a relatively novel technology. The second part is that the health service takes a view of its financial commitments on a year-by-year basis. Even if we can demonstrate that the lifetime cost of putting people with type 1 diabetes onto insulin pumps is 20 percent lower than the cost of healthcare for people on injections, the health service will only view the benefit on a year-by-year basis.

> ## TIP
>
> For those in the UK who are interested in pump therapy, I would advise that you contact a charity called INPUT Diabetes, which provides a fantastic patient advocacy service and helps people with diabetes to gain access to appropriate medical technologies. When I decided that I wanted an insulin pump, the help given to me by John Davis, the founder of INPUT Diabetes, was invaluable. John has now retired, but the charity continues and is run by Lesley Jordan.

Hypos

Have you ever wondered why people with diabetes who use insulin are particularly susceptible to hypos, whilst people without diabetes suffer from them only very occasionally and usually in a very mild form? The answer has many facets, but in simple terms, in a non-diabetic person insulin secreted from the pancreas has a life of 12–15 minutes. Rapidly acting insulin when injected or infused typically takes 10–15 minutes to become active, reaches peak performance in two to three hours, and takes about four hours to clear the system. So whilst we replace our insulin it can never mimic the action profile of innately produced insulin.

Injected insulin has a much longer action profile than natural insulin. We also have another disadvantage in terms of preventing our blood glucose levels from falling too low. The normal response to falling blood glucose levels or low blood glucose levels is to release another hormone from the pancreas called glucagon. It promotes the breakdown of glycogen from the liver, which makes glucose available in the blood, and therefore to the cells of the body. Unfortunately, excess insulin inhibits the breakdown of glycogen, and consequently, our response to falling blood glucose levels is impaired by the very insulin that we inject to keep us alive. As a result, we are at risk of hypoglycaemia. Perhaps this threat will disappear at some point in the future when insulin pumps are used in conjunction with very rapidly acting insulins, having a life that is similar to innately produced insulin of 12–15 minutes. For the time being, at least, we must accept that hypos are just part of life with diabetes and we must be prepared to treat them when they occur.

In my own experience the very best strategy for treating a hypo is to avoid it altogether. My reasoning is that a hypo feels awful and, for some hours after a hypo, I struggle to complete normal daily functions well since my concentration levels are severely impaired. In addition to this it is normal for the body to produce a number of responses to a hypo. We have already discussed the glucagon-glycogen response above, but, in addition to this, the adrenal glands will produce adrenaline (epinephrine), which will stimulate the muscle cells to utilise the glycogen that they have stored, ready for a flight or fight response. The anterior pituitary gland will secrete cortisol, a hormone which makes you resistant to insulin. The result of this cocktail of hormones is that your blood glucose levels will increase. However, the effect of cortisol and adrenaline may take some hours to wear off, and for this reason, high blood glucose levels after a hypo must be managed very conservatively indeed.

Once you have had a hypo you are more likely to experience another hypo in the next 48 hours, because once the store of glycogen has been released from the liver and the muscles there is a debt to be repaid. At random points in the next 48 hours, and with a tendency to happen at night in my own experience, the debt will be repaid as the muscle cells and the liver build glycogen stores again when the plasma glucose is available. Therefore, if you are experiencing hypos, the very best treatment is always to treat the immediate emergency first, but then to run you blood glucose levels a little higher for the next 48 hours. If you use a pump, this might mean a five percent or even ten percent reduction in your basal insulin, and if you use multiple daily injections, it might mean reducing your short-acting acting insulin or eating a modest amount of additional carbohydrates, which you don't administer insulin for over the next couple of days (obviously this depends very much on the dose that you are taking and your body mass).

We have already discussed that hypos are caused because we have too much insulin, but how should we treat a hypo?

A lot of people have their own personal strategy: Many use chocolate, some use jam sandwiches, others use jelly babies or fruit juice and some claim that bananas are the key. In truth, the key to treating a hypo is to use the most rapidly absorbing sugar that you can get. There are hypo treatment gels that are absorbed through the gums and cheeks but personally I find the taste and texture disgusting, although I understand that many people like them. My own preference is to use dextrose tablets, which are cheap to purchase, easy to carry and taste awful – this means that I am never tempted to snack on them when I am hungry! I normally consume 16 grams of glucose via dextrose and then wait for about 20 minutes. If my blood glucose levels have not risen I give another 16 grams of dextrose. If they have risen and remain below target I treat conservatively with a couple of dextrose tablets. In this way I tend to prevent the huge post-hypo glucose spikes that I experience if I use chocolate, for example. I also tend to prevent myself from getting the post-hypo munchies, which would have me attacking the grocery store like a swarm of locusts devouring everything in sight. This would feel great for a while until my blood glucose levels began to rise, and rise, and rise. When treating a hypo it is essential to make sure that you are well hydrated. A fluid deficit will slow down the absorption of glucose.

Finally, you should note that recent studies by Dr Alistair Lumb (www.runsweet.org) have demonstrated that, when you are hypo, a very quick and effective strategy to raise blood glucose levels is to do a 20–30 second maximum speed sprint. This appears to utilise the glycogen stored in muscle cells to raise blood glucose levels. You should still continue to treat the hypo as appropriate, but this might be a useful strategy for those times when you don't have any glucose on you. Of course, this never happens to any of us, does it? I can't wait to try this one when I am sitting in a large corporate office and my blood glucose levels drop, the looks on the faces of the people around me are guaranteed to be priceless.

High Blood Glucose Levels (Hyperglycaemia)

Treating high blood glucose levels or hyperglycaemia is an art form all of its own. The natural temptation is to give a large dose of insulin to bring blood glucose levels down quickly. It is widely accepted that the higher your blood glucose level, the more resistant you become to insulin, and many of us can remember being in Diabetic Ketoacidosis, which we want to avoid at all costs. However, giving large doses of insulin can cause its own problems, since it might take a while to get blood glucose levels moving in the right direction. My own experience is once they start falling, they tend to continue falling and rapidly. If an infection or illness is the cause of the high blood glucose levels, you may see sustained high blood glucose levels for a few days or even weeks until the infection is brought under control. When I used multiple daily injections I would typically increase my short-acting insulin to deal with high blood glucose levels, since it takes several days for the long-acting insulin to have an effect. Just be aware that, if the high blood glucose levels are not caused by illness or an exceptional event like eating a large meal, etc., it might be that the long-acting insulin needs adjusting. These days on the insulin pump it is much easier to deal with this as I can give corrections on the pump and set temporary increases to my basal (background) insulin. As with everything else in diabetes management, conservative management techniques are usually the best.

TIP

If my blood glucose is 13.1mmol/l (236 mg/dL) or more, I give a correction dose of 10% of my normal total daily insulin dose and drink 200ml of water every half hour.

If my blood glucose is 17.0mmol/l (306mg/dL) or more, I give a correction dose of 20% of my normal total daily dose and drink 200ml of water every half hour.

Before taking any insulin or action, it is ESSENTIAL that I understand why my blood glucose levels are high. If it is the result of eating a pizza and my carbohydrate and insulin absorption rates don't match, there is little to worry about, but the CRITICAL thing is to make sure that I don't already have loads of insulin already administered that will deal with this. Personal judgement and experience are essential here.

Before I was able to get an insulin pump I had to do a training course called 'Dose Adjustment for Normal Eating' (DAfNE), and the strategies that it taught for dealing with high blood glucose levels were wonderful.

These metrics seem to work well for me: I'll always check my blood glucose an hour after giving a correction. If my blood glucose is the same or has lowered, my shot was effective. If my blood glucose has continued to rise, more insulin is required and I need to investigate the reason for my high blood glucose. Was it due to consumed carbohydrates that I forgot to give insulin for? Is my pump working? Has my insulin gone off? Do I have an infection? At this point I get fresh insulin from the fridge and I give another correction dose of rapid-acting insulin, using a syringe or Novopen. An hour later I check my blood glucose levels again, and if they have continued to rise, I can already discount a fault with my pump or insulin as the cause.

I typically find that, when my diabetes management needs improvement, there are a number of key areas that I can focus on to quickly gain good management and I have put them into simple bullet points below.

- **Most diabetes management issues are caused by too much insulin.** If I notice a long-term control problem, the first thing I usually do is drop my daily dose of insulin by 10 percent, which prevents hypos and subsequent rebound high blood glucose levels. Over the next few days, I then make careful records and adjustments to my insulin levels. It is easier to bring high blood glucose levels down slowly over a few days, than to keep reacting to high and low blood glucose levels.

- Most of my diabetes management challenges are resolved when my background or basal levels of insulin are right. Testing basal insulin levels is tedious but always worth it.

- Avoid low blood glucose levels. It really is OK to run blood glucose levels high for a few days and bring them down conservatively, but remember high blood glucose levels are OK provided that they are not causing DKA and they are limited to only a few days.

- When bringing high blood glucose levels down, don't aim to get to target levels instantly. This would involve taking a relatively large dose of insulin, which could lead to a hypo.

- Unless I have a dangerously high blood glucose level, I allow at least four hours between each bolus of insulin. This prevents the stacking of insulin, which would cause my blood glucose level to drop too far and too fast.

- Be aware of Dr Bernstein's law of small numbers. The accuracy of blood glucose measurements is +/- 20%, the accuracy of nutrition information is +/-20%, and the repeatability of injecting the same dose of insulin into the same patient in the same location can vary by up to 39 percent. By keeping the amount of carbohydrates consumed low and the doses of insulin low, you reduce the significance of all of this variability, and you improve your diabetes management.

- The value of a single blood glucose measurement is limited. The real value is in the pattern of blood glucose that we observe, and good records or a continuous glucose meter are valuable tools in recognising these patterns. Good diabetes management comes from being proactive in dealing with the pattern, not from being reactive; in other words, take the actions necessary to avoid the low and high blood glucose levels before they occur.

Dawn Phenomenon and the Symogi Effect

Waking up in the morning with consistently high blood glucose levels could have multiple causes, but broadly the two main candidates are the dawn phenomenon and the Symogi effect. The result of both of these issues is identical: You wake with a high blood glucose level. It is usually seen on a consistent basis, and, of course, the natural reaction to a high blood glucose level is to give more insulin at that time. If we see this as a consistent pattern we could be forgiven for increasing our overnight background insulin.

Dawn phenomenon occurs in just about everybody when your body is in a deep sleep state. A part of your brain, called the reticular arousal system, brings you from a sleep state to a conscious state in the morning. One of the mechanisms it uses to do this is to promote the release of a hormone called cortisol, which makes you insulin resistant. The reticular arousal system is also considered to promote the release of catecholamines, which also make you insulin resistant, although the precise mechanism of catecholamines in the sleep-wake cycle is still poorly understood. We understand enough about cortisol and catecholamines to know that they increase our blood glucose levels by making us resistant to insulin. This is a normal reaction in all people, not just people with diabetes. The challenge that it presents for us is that we need additional active insulin available in the hours between about 03:00 a.m. and 10:00 a.m., but if we are using a shot of long-acting insulin at bedtime the action profile is flat. We can minimise the effect of dawn phenomenon, but we are then at an increased risk of hypoglycaemia throughout the day, as the cortisol and catecholamines effects wear off.

The Symogi effect is quite different. When you have a hypo the body responds by producing and releasing glucagon, which in turn releases glycogen from the liver and has a massive cascade effect on raising the blood glucose levels. This is part of the body's natural defence system against low blood glucose levels. If a hypo is occurring as you sleep and remains untreated glycogen will be released to reverse the hypo; in addition to this, you will be releasing adrenaline (epinephrine), and you will wake up the next morning with a high blood glucose level. Treating this with insulin needs to be done with caution, because you are now very sensitive to insulin and you have a massively increased risk of a hypo over the next two to three days as the liver (and muscles) restores glycogen supplies at random times. If you wake each morning with a high blood glucose level, you could be forgiven for increasing the night time background insulin, but this would only increase the severity of night time hypos and make things worse.

If you are waking each morning with high blood glucose levels, the only way you can resolve it is by working out if it is a result of the dawn phenomenon or the Symogi effect, perform a blood glucose measurement before the hormones associated with the wake cycle are released. This means that you need blood glucose data between 02:00 and 03:00 in the morning. If these numbers indicate hypoglycaemia, the Symogi effect is to blame and less overnight insulin is required, and if they are not suggestive of hypoglycaemia, the dawn phenomenon is the most likely cause, so more overnight insulin is required. It does not matter how much I know about diabetes and the good reasons why these measurements are necessary, I still hate the 02:00 a.m. blood glucose measurements!

CHAPTER EIGHT

GLUCOSE MONITORING

If you have read the chapters in this book in sequence you have gained a lot of knowledge about diabetes and about some of the ways in which it can and will affect your life. You have seen how, as a community and as individuals, we work 24 hours a day, 7 days a week, 52 weeks of the year for every single year of our lives. There is no other job like it: You get no thanks, no pay, and no holiday. It is easy to get depressed. However, it is time to turn all of that around.

Living with diabetes is always going to be a challenge. You can either accept the challenge, or you can pretend that the challenge will go away. It will not. At least not until some of the brilliant scientists who are working on our behalf find a way to cure diabetes. It is your responsibility now to do something to become engaged in your diabetes: You need the tools to empower yourself to achieve your goals today, tomorrow, and for the rest of your life.

We need to start talking about monitoring blood glucose levels. It is essential that you gather good data because it will empower you to make informed decisions on the best way to treat your current diabetes challenge in this moment. I love to see what my blood glucose levels are because I am able to make some predictions about the next few hours, and I can quickly and easily modify my carbohydrates or my insulin, so that I can do whatever I want. The value of measuring my blood glucose levels is huge, but when I make careful records about my blood glucose levels, and I take time to review those records some surprising patterns can and do emerge, these are priceless. For many years I was using a spreadsheet that I developed to record my blood glucose levels and it was brilliant. The problem for me is that I am great at taking my blood glucose measurements. I am great at acting on the results, but I find taking the time and motivation to record and review my results is the difficult part.

TIP

For me, personally, when my blood glucose levels are recorded and I review the patterns and make informed treatment decisions, my HbA1c is at least 15% lower than when I simply take blood glucose measurements. The Diabetes Control and Complications Trial (DCCT) (1992) teaches us that for every 10% reduction in HbA1c there is a 35% reduction in the risks of developing secondary symptoms of diabetes including retinopathy. There is no doubt in my mind that the more data I have and the better I am able to observe the patterns that occur, the better I feel and the better my diabetes is managed.

Things are getting a lot easier with today's technology because many people now have smart phones, android tablets, and iPads, and there is a variety of software available out there for recording blood glucose levels. I have tried many, and my personal favourite is one called MySugr. One of the reasons that it is so outstanding is that the team that set up MySugr and developed the product all have type 1 diabetes and they are passionate about helping people with diabetes. There are even versions for children, which enable the parent to see the results as they are recorded. The application also allows children to take photos of food, which can be shared with a parent or caregiver, so that they can get assistance in estimating carbohydrate content. All this can happen even when parents and caregivers are miles away from their children. In addition to all of this, the reports it produces are exceptionally clear and well formatted because they have been developed by people who understand what a person with diabetes really needs.

Blood glucose monitoring has become very quick, almost pain free, and is easy to do. The more information that we have about our own diabetes and how it responds to the challenges we face, the more empowered we are to do something about those challenges. So how often should we measure our blood glucose levels? In my opinion, at a minimum, we should all be measuring our blood glucose on waking in the morning, before each meal (which for many people translates to before each shot of insulin). We should also measure our blood glucose any time that we feel something is not quite right and before exercise. If you have exercised you will also need to measure your blood glucose immediately after exercise and, ideally, again at 8 and 12 hours post exercise. In addition to this, if you live in the UK and you drive a vehicle, the Driver and Vehicle Licencing Authority (DVLA) has a legal requirement that you measure your blood glucose 45 minutes before driving, and that you stop and test every two hours whilst driving. To put it simply, you need to measure your blood glucose often. I know that the rules on driving differ in other parts of the world.

Many of us with type 1 diabetes have in recent years had some difficulty in obtaining an appropriate number of blood glucose strips because these strips are expensive. If you are testing eight and ten times a day, which many of us are, you will get through in the region of 200–300 blood glucose strips each month. This is not unusual in people who want optimum management of their diabetes. After my own prescription to blood glucose strips was restricted a few years ago, and I managed to get this decision reversed, I decided that I would write an article for INPUT Diabetes to help others facing this situation. You can get the full version with the hyperlinks here at www.inputdiabetes.org.uk/glucose-monitoring/access-to-test-strips/. I have also included a copy of the text here:

Access to blood glucose test strips

Has your GP changed the quantity or type of blood glucose test strips that you get on prescription – without asking you? If so, you're not alone.

Across the UK, Clinical Commissioning Groups (CCGs) (in England) and Local Health Boards (in Scotland & Wales) are attempting to reduce the cost of diabetes care by limiting the number of blood glucose test strips available on prescription. Some authorities are requiring people with diabetes to use a particular blood glucose meter so they can buy strips in bulk at lower prices.

Saving money within the NHS should be encouraged, provided that the changes needed are consistent with National Institute for Clinical Excellence (NICE) guidelines and clinical evidence. NICE Clinical Guidance 15 'Diagnosis and management of type 1 diabetes in children, young people and adults' says:

1.2.6.9: **Children and young people** with type 1 diabetes and their families **should be offered a choice** of appropriate equipment for undertaking monitoring of capillary blood glucose to optimise their glycaemic control in response to adjustment of insulin, diet and exercise.

and

1.8.2.4: Self monitoring should be performed using meters and strips **chosen by adults** with diabetes **to suit their needs**, and usually with low blood requirements, fast analysis times and integral memories. (INPUT's emphasis)

Yet in many cases, individuals' needs and preferences have not been taken into account. This tendency to discount patients as stakeholders needs to be addressed in order to maintain and improve the quality of diabetes care in the UK.

Patient Choice in Blood Glucose Testing

In July 2012, the Department of Health published a consultation document called 'Liberating the

NHS: No decision about me, without me', which has been endorsed by the Secretary of State for Health. As the title suggests, healthcare providers need to engage in dialogue with patients regarding treatments to meet individual needs. On the other side of the coin, we as patients need to engage in a long-term partnership with respect to our health. You have a right to feel satisfied that you have had adequate consultation and reached an agreement with your healthcare provider, rather than being told what to do.

Obtaining Adequate Glucose Testing Strips

It has often been said that 99% of diabetes care is self-care: Many people with type 1 diabetes spend less than 24 hours in the company of diabetes care professionals in an average year. Patients' ability to self-manage diabetes depends on access to appropriate resources, including both drugs and blood glucose monitoring.

If your GP does not give you adequate test strips on the grounds of cost, this simple statement may be all you need to persuade them: 'If you think test strips are expensive, wait until you see how much it costs when I don't test.'

If that argument doesn't work, you could try the following steps in order:

1.   Discuss the matter with your GP. Even though it might seem obvious, say you have

type 1 diabetes and have different needs from someone with type 2 diabetes.

2. Print this article, and this letter, and discuss them with your GP.

3. Ask your diabetes consultant or diabetes specialist nurse to write to the GP to explain your individual clinical needs with regard to blood glucose testing.

4. Raise the matter with your CCG/Local Health Board. Your GP will be able to give you the relevant contact information. In many parts of the country, local policies do not distinguish between type 1 and type 2 diabetes.

5. Contact your local MP and ask them to help you resolve the situation.

If you would like support in following these steps, consider contacting a patient advocacy organisation. INPUT, JDRF and Diabetes UK are all taking an active interest in access to blood glucose testing and may be able to assist you.

Driving and Blood Glucose Testing

In addition to the long-standing minimum clinical requirements, since January 2012 the DVLA has made it mandatory for all people who use insulin and hold a driving licence to test blood glucose levels before driving and every 2 hours whilst driving. The current DVLA driving licence application form states:

'You MUST sign the declaration that you will test before and every two hours when you drive. [This is to let the DVLA know that you understand that you have to test while driving.] This is a legal requirement and a licence will not be issued if this declaration is not signed.'

People who use insulin must have access to an appropriate number of blood glucose test strips to be safe on the road. If your GP has reduced your test strip prescription so that you don't have enough strips to comply with the DVLA rules, it is very important to push back! Your life and others' safety may depend on it.

TIP

Your health and your life depend upon appropriate access to insulin, medical supplies, and technologies. If you are not happy with the service that you are receiving at any point, stop and reflect upon the situation, asking yourself and your healthcare team, 'How can I gain access to the essential supplies and advice that I need to keep me alive and healthy?'.

Continuous Glucose Monitors (CGM)

When we perform blood glucose measurements we gain great information but even when we diligently record this information it provides us with a small data set. We can see perhaps eight or ten moments in our day, which inform our decisions about our diabetes management. For many of us with diabetes we are pretty good at measuring our blood glucose levels, but what is happening in that overnight period? We might not be eating and drinking, but a whole variety of physiological changes happen as we sleep and wake. When I wake in the morning, if my blood glucose levels are too low from a nighttime hypo, I am exhausted before I even get out of bed.

If my blood glucose levels are high I wake up feeling like I have the flu. Whilst it is easy to treat a high blood glucose level, it still takes a couple of hours for my blood glucose levels to return to normal levels. The issue is not in how I feel at that moment or in treating the high blood glucose with additional insulin, but in understanding why my blood glucose level is high. Is it because my background (basal) insulin levels are too low? Is it because of food that I ate yesterday evening that I gave the wrong amount of insulin for? Is it that the food I ate last night had a high fat and carbohydrate content, like pizza or Chinese food, which typically causes the absorption of carbohydrates to be delayed for a few hours? This would mean that my insulin action profile and the food absorption were mismatched. Is it because I have an infection? Is it because I had a hypo in the night? Or, is it because I am suffering from dawn phenomenon? Remember this is the process of cortisol and adrenaline making me insulin resistant in the predawn to mid-morning hours. Without good data, it is difficult to determine why this has happened and, although I can treat it reactively, gaining greater management of my diabetes means that I need to treat these episodes proactively. I need to prevent them in the first place, and to do this, I need to record and identify the patterns in my blood glucose levels.

Continuous Glucose Monitors (CGM) are devices about the same size as an insulin pump and, in fact, some insulin pumps are already equipped with the CGM receivers built in. They work by measuring the concentration of the glucose in between the cells, typically in the subcutaneous tissues. A small needle introduces a sensor into the skin and the needle is taken out, leaving the very fine sensor wires behind. The sensor wires typically stay in for about a week and are connected to a transmitter, which sends the information to a remote receiver. The systems typically take a glucose measurement every five minutes and send them to the receiver, and you get to see information about what is happening throughout the whole day and night. I have tried two systems, one from Medtronic and the other from Dexcom, and both provided me with valuable insights. Personally, I found the sensors for the Medtronic system a little uncomfortable and not nearly as accurate as the Dexcom system. But I am willing to admit this may have been user error.

CGM technology is truly incredible, but because they measure the fluid between the cells (interstitial fluid) and not the blood, there is a delay of about 15 minutes between the CGM results and blood glucose testing. The systems need to be calibrated against blood glucose measurements a couple of times each day, even so, there can still be discrepancies between CGM readings and blood glucose measurements. For these reasons CGM cannot be used to make instant treatment decisions, and you still need to perform blood glucose tests to inform your treatment. The value of CGM is on seeing the patterns and trends of what is actually happening in every single minute of the day and night.

We are currently in the same position with CGM that we were at in the 1980s with the self-monitoring of blood glucose levels. Clinically, the data that CGM provides is essential to gaining fantastic control; however in the UK, the cost of these devices is prohibitive to the health service. Until the National Institute of Clinical Excellence (NICE) performs a technology appraisal on these devices showing that they improve patient outcomes, they are not likely to be offered widely on the National Health Service. NICE has no concerns about improving the quality of a patient's life as they are only concerned with acting as financial guardians to the NHS. What does this mean for us? Once again, we have a situation where technology is available to massively improve patient outcomes but, until we get data that shows these systems help us to minimise the costs to the NHS, they remain a largely self-funded option.

The cost of CGM systems is high; they have an initial start up cost in excess of £1,000 to purchase the transmitter and receiver, although this might be considerably less if your insulin pump already has a receiver built in. The life of the transmitter is limited by the life of the battery in the transmitter. For some devices these are rechargeable; for others, these are long-life batteries that last for about a year, but whatever system you have the transmitter will need periodic replacement. As I write this paragraph I just ordered a replacement transmitter for my own CGM this morning. My transmitter has lasted for 11 months and was in almost constant use in this period. However, the major cost of a CGM system is, without doubt, the cost of the sensors themselves. These cost around £60 for each sensor, and a sensor is licensed to last for about a week. In my experience of using a Medtronic system for about eight weeks, I found the sensors which were designed to last for six days were struggling to last for the duration. However, the Dexcom sensors are licensed for seven days, and as they expire, I simply restart the sensor. On average, I am able to extend the life of a sensor from seven days to about nineteen days in this way, and typically they only fail as the adhesive on the sensor wears off. I have heard stories of people making a sensor last for forty-two days. Extending the life on sensors reduces the cost of running a CGM system considerably.

The cost of running a CGM system is high, but the value of the data I get from my CGM is worth every penny, and my health and well-being has improved massively since investing in my CGM system. I appreciate that the cost of CGM may be beyond the reach of many people, but if there is any way that you can possibly afford it, I urge you to consider this for the benefit of your health. If you simply cannot afford a CGM, ask your hospital to loan you a CGM system for a limited period of time; most clinics are happy to do this to help you resolve a control issue. If you need to, tell the hospital that you suspect that you are having hypos as you sleep at night and you are not waking to treat them. The symptoms of this could be normal blood glucose levels at bedtime and low blood glucose levels before or about 03:00 a.m., and you will wake up with high blood glucose levels. I am sure that any decent diabetes centre will be eager to help you resolve this issue, and CGM is the best tool we have for the job right now.

The Artificial Pancreas

Medtronic recently released a new insulin pump in the USA, technically it is called the 530g. However, they are marketing it as an artficial pancreas. I am sorry to report that in my opinion nothing could be further from the truth. The 530g is similar to the Medtronic Veo pump, which has been available in Europe for a few years now and could not get licensed by the FDA in the USA. This pump is remarkable technology and has an in-built CGM receiver and when used with the Medtronic CGM sensors and transmitter the pump will suspend insulin delivery for a couple of hours if a hypo is identified and not treated. Normal basal insulin delivery starts automatically after two hours. The advantage of this system is that untreated night time hypoglycaemia is no longer a huge worry.

A true artificial pancreas will provide us with a closed loop system that can monitor our glucose levels, giving insulin and glucagon in response to changing blood glucose levels to maintain normal glycemic control, without needing to worry about ensuring that the pump is preprogrammed to deliver the right amount of basal insulin at the right time. It will also take care of giving insulin in response to food eaten without the requirement for user intervention. The great news is that clinical trials of this system are already happening now and if the trials are as promising as the initial results reported by JDRF, I believe that we will see this system reaching the market quite soon.

CHAPTER NINE

THE CHALLENGES

Anybody who has lived with diabetes has probably heard the horror stories about the complications that can occur in poorly controlled diabetes. I have found that many people in my life have tried to use these complications as leverage to inspire me to improve my control. For me this is never going to work and, as far as I can tell from other people that I know who have diabetes, it does not seem to work for them either. Managing your diabetes from a perspective of fear and avoidance is never going to motivate and inspire you.

First let us talk about the correct language with this disorder, since there are no complications to diabetes – there are only secondary symptoms. Secondary symptoms are conditions that are associated with diabetes and they typically occur after many years of living with it. These days we are increasingly seeing reports in the media about the cost of diabetes care and the burden of diabetes care on the healthcare system. Let us make something absolutely clear here, the figures that get quoted encompass all types of diabetes. Remember that type 2 diabetes is typically diagnosed in older people who are already presenting to their healthcare providers with other health issues and that type 2 diabetes accounts for 90 percent of all cases of diabetes.

Each year Diabetes UK produces a report called 'State of the

Nation', which reviews the performance of diabetes care across the UK. In all honesty, it is a politically motivated report, which is aimed at policy makers in the various healthcare systems. I think the report is a great tool and it focuses on the fifteen essential healthcare checks that people with diabetes must expect, but if you decide to read it, please do remember that the report is written in a negative way to engage the healthcare system to address their failings according to Diabetes UK. The organisation has a tendency to focus on type 2 diabetes, because this represents the majority of their membership base. I will quote these words from the 2013 edition of the report:

> *People with diabetes also run a greater risk of developing one or more severe health complications, which can greatly impact on their independence, quality of life and economic contribution. Many of these complications are avoidable. With good risk assessment and early diagnosis, patient education, support and good ongoing care, they need not happen.*

We could spend considerable time here talking about the complications but if we did that this book would become like every other publication on diabetes. I have already been treated and continue to be treated for diabetic retinopathy, but it is still my belief that we have three powerful tools against diabetes and its secondary symptoms:

Positive mindset. Your emotions are yours to own and run. It is up to you to decide how you are going to feel in any single moment; find ways to put yourself into a positive mental state and visit that place often. Remember you are not in this alone;

your family, friends and loved ones are part of this journey too. You must find a support network that works well for you, so if there is not one out there, create one.

Blood Pressure. Maintaining a low blood pressure helps to protect us from many of the secondary symptoms of diabetes. The longer that you have had diabetes the more challenging maintaining a low blood pressure can become due to damage to the kidneys and to the blood vessels. If your blood pressure is elevated, take action to bring it down. This might be taking ACE inhibitors or ACE-II Antagonists, which prevent vasodilation and lower blood pressure. Having fantastic nutrition and regular cardiovascular exercise will certainly help in this part of the process.

The Holy Grail of maintaining blood glucose levels that are close to normal non-diabetic levels will be of enormous benefit. The great thing here is that no matter how long you have been diabetic, you can always improve your diabetes management. Most secondary symptoms respond positively, and some even abate when glycemic management is good.

Living with Diabetes

I decided early on that diabetes was going to adjust to my life, instead of the other way around, and that diabetes would not stop me doing the things I wanted to do. In truth this was a lie I told myself, since my diabetes has shaped me into the person I am today. Almost everything that I do and every decision I make reflects back to how my diabetes will respond to that situation, and what mitigations I need to take.

We cannot complete this journey of living with diabetes

without looking at some of the factors that will impact our diabetes and the management of diabetes. Going to school with diabetes was not particularly difficult for me, but for my parents I suspect it was much harder. There were isolated incidents when teachers had failed to understand my needs as a person with diabetes and I recall a teacher giving me a lunch time detention that delayed my lunch by 45 minutes one day, which led to a hypo.

As a teenager my diabetes management was nonexistent. I exercised regularly, but I paid no attention to my nutrition and even less to my blood glucose management. I am not alone with this part of my journey if you investigate the age distributed HbA1c results for the population of people with diabetes the highest readings occurring between the ages of 17 and 26. This is exactly consistent with my own journey, and during this time, college, university, and independent living all occur for most people. College and university, in particular, are challenging environments because of the lack of a day-to-day routine. Having six hours of consecutive lectures one day, an 08:00 a.m. start the next, and an 11:00 a.m. start the following day make finding patterns in blood glucose management challenging. In addition to all of this suddenly you are cooking or not cooking for yourself; you may have a very limited budget for food, and the temptation to drink alcohol in your new found freedom can be high.

The advent of multiple daily injections made dealing with the variable daily routine in college and university easier. One of my friends from university also has type 1 diabetes, and he had a really tough time, regularly needing help from the paramedics as his flat mates could not wake him in the mornings. Luckily he had great flat mates.

Alcohol

In my teens and early twenties I never could get used to drinking beer, it always made me feel really bloated, even after just a pint. It was many years before I discovered that I have Coeliacs disease, which means that gluten, found in wheat, barley, and rye (this includes beer hops), causes an immune response in my gut. This was probably fortunate in that it stopped me from drinking large amounts and I never really developed a taste for spirits or cider.

The issue for people with diabetes is that most alcohol contains significant amounts of sugar but alcohol itself lowers blood glucose levels. As a person with type 1 diabetes you will get drunk on considerably less alcohol volume than somebody who does not have diabetes. Alcohol lowers your blood glucose levels, and the risk of becoming hypoglycaemic is increased for about 12–16 hours after you stop drinking. Hypoglycaemia and drunken behaviour are almost identical, so if you are hypo and drunk, how will people tell the difference and who is going to help you to treat your hypo? Alcohol lowers your inhibitions, and for me, when I consume alcohol, I usually end the evening with my body craving carbohydrates, to which I usually succumb. This is probably a protection mechanism to deal with and prevent hypoglycaemia, but the results are usually very high blood glucose levels the following morning. The decision to drink alcohol is a personal one, and you must be comfortable with the people around you, who must know about your diabetes and have the ability to deal with your hypoglycaemia, even if they are drunk themselves. Personally, I don't touch alcohol unless I am with people that I can trust implicitly with my life, not only in the time that I am drinking, but also in the 12–16 hours afterwards.

> **TIP**
>
> It is OK to drink alcohol in moderation, but know the risks it presents and have an action plan of how you are going to deal with them when they become issues. The people you drink and live with really might need to save your life, make sure that you can trust them, and that you have their consent that they are happy and willing to help you. You cannot afford to assume that they can and will help you, when you have passed out after drinking 10 pints of beer.

School, College, and University

I have only a distant memory of how my diabetes impacted me at school, but I can remember that special provisions were made for me in the school kitchens. The school cooks would work with my mother each day to make sure that my meal contained the right portion of carbohydrates. I can also remember that I had special provision to eat my lunch at a particular time, regardless of whether my class had the early or late lunch setting. Beyond this, I don't really remember a great deal of difference between me and the other children that I grew up with. Of course, I was only five-years-old at diagnosis, so I cannot compare my experiences of school pre- and post-diabetes.

Schools now are required to have an individual education plan which accommodates a child with diabetes and their special needs to have insulin in the school and for dextrose to be available whenever it is required. I suspect that for very young children somebody in the school would need to be trained in how to measure blood glucose levels, so that appropriate action can be taken. However, it is essential for parents to educate the school or ask their diabetes specialist nurses to educate the school. Teachers are typically not trained in diabetes and most have little or no experience of dealing with it. Mistakes will be made, and it is easy to get angry at education providers for these errors, but the best route is to teach them how to do a better job next time. Rather than complain about this reflect upon how much knowledge you had about diabetes before it became part of your life.

College and university are going to be challenging times for anybody with type 1 diabetes, because the hours are irregular and the day-to-day routine does not exist in the same way as at home. Multiple daily injections are invaluable here, but in my opinion, the best strategy for this stage of life is to use an insulin pump because it gives you maximum freedom. The biggest part of the challenge at this phase is typically age related; we have already discussed how diabetes management is at its poorest levels in the late teens and early twenties. I believe that psychological counselling needs to be offered to everybody who lives with diabetes, so that they can come to terms with their diabetes and they can challenge their diabetes in positive ways, rather than to keep trying to be like everybody else whilst denying the importance of their diabetes. This counseling should be available to everybody living with diabetes not just the person with diabetes.

Work and Careers

In the UK, type 1 diabetes is covered by the Disability Discrimination Act (DDA), which classifies it as a hidden disability. This means that your employer is not allowed to discriminate against you on terms that you have diabetes. However, should you tell your employer that you have diabetes? If so, when should you tell them? The strategy that I have typically found that works the best for me is to wait until an employment offer is made before disclosing that I have diabetes and will need to take appropriate time to manage the condition, so it doesn't interfere with my performance. If the employment offer is suddenly withdrawn the employer is breaking the law, since you have now informed them of your needs and stated that you expect your performance to be equal to everybody else's. We know that there will be times when this is simply not true; for example, if you are hypo and taking the time to treat a hypo so that you can continue to perform at work, it means that you will be excelling in your chosen activities again very quickly, although not as soon as a non-diabetic person.

I see people posting on social media sites asking what job their son or daughter with diabetes can do. Please don't ask this question. Remember never to tell your children that they can't be whatever they want to be (if they are diabetic or not) when they grow up. It is a mistake. Not because they can't, but because it would never have occurred to them they couldn't! A better question might be how can my daughter with type 1 diabetes be the first woman to walk on the moon, join the army, be an airline pilot, or whatever else it is that she has decided to do? The boundaries to the professions that we can take are limited by our own beliefs, certainly there are some jobs that we cannot do for the safety of ourselves and others. Never make assumptions, always investigate and understand the issues. I know an engineer with type 1 diabetes who works at a nuclear power station, his job takes him into radiation contaminated zones around the reactor. He was determined that his insulin pump, which might get a dose of radiation and then would need to be destroyed, would not be a barrier in his career, so he designed and built a metal-shielded box for his insulin pump, protecting it from radiation.

Stress and Illness

Stress and illness typically make your blood glucose levels elevated. It is normal to need a little more insulin to correct for these episodes. It is always OK to adjust your insulin dose, provided that you understand how to do it, and what the effects are likely to be. If you are not sure, please seek medical advice, and remember that conservative corrections are better because you can always add more insulin later but once you have given insulin you cannot take it back.

I encourage everybody to develop a good relationship with their diabetes specialist nurses. They perform a great job and are a great source of expert knowledge and experience. Typically they are only a phone call away and they are experts at recognising the patterns in your blood glucose levels that you had never even thought about. How can they do this? Each day they are looking at hundreds of sets of data, and they see recurring themes very quickly. I have been saved from diabetes disasters and hospital admissions with a little telephone support and my knowledge. My experience of diabetes has been made so much better by the work that these incredible people do.

> ### TIP
>
> Even if you don't attend a diabetes clinic make sure
> that you get a Diabetes Specialist Nurse (DSN),
> in the US and Canada I believe these are called
> Certified Diabetes Educators (CDE's), to help you
> make control decisions when you are not sure how
> to deal with an ongoing diabetes situation. However,
> for all emergencies, you should always seek urgent
> medical advice from your doctor, the paramedics
> or the emergency facilities at your local hospital as
> appropriate.

Diabetes Burnout

Living with type 1 diabetes is hard work, and there is no possibility of a vacation. Even the most diligent people occasionally get tired and they relax their management a little from time to time. I certainly do this since it is one of my coping strategies. Without any doubt, I feel my best when my diabetes is well managed; during that time, I am getting amazing nutrition, and I am getting a lot of cardiovascular exercise. Just like everything else in life, if you can instill great habits for 80 percent of the time, the remaining 20 percent will take care of itself. You can actually afford to eat a bit more or to drink some alcohol or to have a day where you do only a few blood glucose measurements. Your standards for taking care of your health on these 'zag days' will probably still be quite high, and you probably won't go absolutely wild. You will notice that you don't feel so great when your management techniques slip because you are used to feeling well. The danger of these 'zag' days is that the occasional day is fine, but just because you can get away with it for one day, every now and again, does not mean that you can every day. It is incredible how quickly great diabetes management becomes poor diabetes management, and I speak from experience!

What I am trying to say here is that we all need a day or two off from the constant and never-ending measuring and analysing of everything that we eat, drink, do or don't do, and working out how we are going to deal with it. It is OK to do that, and, if you happen to be the loved one of a person with diabetes or the caregiver, please don't judge us for this.

However, from experience I suggest that when you successfully have a relaxed diabetes day and you get away with it, it's easy for that to become two days, and then to turn the days into a week; very quickly, it becomes the new normal. When you are suffering from burnout, find strategies that help you get back on track. Set a day on which you are going to relax your diabetes management and enjoy it, but be sure that you know that normal management starts again tomorrow. Ask family and friends to help you enjoy the moment, and ask for their help in encouraging you to keep to your normal high standards of diabetes management if you need them to. One friend of mine has a night off each week when her husband takes over control of her diabetes management and he measures her blood glucose levels and makes the treatment decisions on her behalf. The great thing about this is that her husband is fully engaged in her diabetes care and if she ever needs his help when she is unwell, he has already practised his strategies for managing her diabetes.

Travel and Flight

Travelling with insulin is relatively easy, but always make sure that, if you are travelling overseas, you have adequate travel insurance, a letter from your healthcare team, explaining why you need to carry drugs and syringes and, of course, adequate supplies for your trip.

On one particularly memorable occasion quite a few years ago, I had been working in Edinburgh for a few days and was flying back home to London. I was carrying only hand luggage, which had a few days of clothes in it, toiletries, my laptop computer, and of course, my insulin. My bag was randomly selected at the X-ray machine for a manual search. Normally I am extremely polite about this and I warn the customs about my insulin and used sharps before they open my bag. On this occasion, the customs guy made the mistake of being rude to me at the outset, and so I kept my mouth shut. When he pulled out my bag containing my diabetes supplies grunted 'What is this?' Deciding to provoke him, I told him it was my drugs. He went pale and told me that he was going to confiscate my drugs on the spot. I told him that he was welcome to do that provided I could have my mobile phone and laptop back. He asked why they were so important, obviously suspecting that they contained an illicit stash, so I told him that I needed to connect to the Internet in order to get phone numbers for all of the national daily newspapers to tell them how the UK customs agency confiscated life-saving insulin from a person with type 1 diabetes. His attitude changed instantly and, after confirming my claims, he let me thorough customs. This strategy is not to be recommended, but I have to admit I did enjoy his reaction.

I confess that whenever I fly my routine for diabetes management is usually destroyed, and it takes me a day or two to bring my blood glucose levels back to normal. This is especially true on long-haul travelling, where you are waking at odd hours and being fed airline food that you have no control over at bizarre hours of the day and night. I typically find that, whenever I can, I prefer to make my own arrangements for food on flights; on a short haul this is easy, as I don't eat, but it is more challenging on a long haul. A strategy that has recently been suggested is to disconnect the pump during take off and landing. Evidence suggests that air bubbles can form in the pump tubing as aircraft pressure changes. I have not tried this yet but the physics behind this appear to make sense. You may need to prime the air out of the tubing before you reconnect!

When it comes to changing insulin to comply with different time zones, I have found that the best way to do this is to change my wristwatch and insulin pump settings to the time zone of the destination point at the moment that I sit down on the plane. This means that I need to be extra vigilant about my blood glucose levels and I often need to take corrections of either glucose or insulin during a long-haul flight. If you are using a basal-bolus injection regime and travelling long haul, many doctors now recommend that you do not give the basal insulin on the day that you fly, but instead use short-acting insulin every four to six hours until you are safely back into a normal 24-hour day cycle. In many ways this emulates what I would do with an insulin pump, but always ask for advice and work out your strategy before travelling.

If you use an insulin pump and/or a continuous glucose monitor, under no circumstances should they pass throughout the X-ray scanner at the airport. Keep them on you at all times, and ask customs to perform a manual search of you. If customs asks to see where the insulin pump or cgm transmitters are located, it is not unreasonable for you to ask for this to be carried out in privacy. One final word of caution, most of the time, I find that the customs people are great at doing a manual search, but every now and then, they can be very heavy handed and one actually managed to dislodge my pump set when he pulled it so hard. Therefore, before the manual search begins, remind them that these devices are connected to you on the inside, and it hurts when they are disturbed. Ask them to be as gentle as possible and always remain polite, since they are only doing their job and keeping us all safe.

Dating and Intimacy

You don't have to tell a prospective or new girlfriend or boyfriend that you have diabetes straight away, but if you are going out on a few dates and you are eating at restaurants and/or are drinking alcohol, it is in your best interest to inform them early. Make them aware that if your personality suddenly changes randomly, it is not because you are a crazed psychopath, but that you might need to test your blood glucose levels and take some dextrose.

If the relationship develops into an intimate one and you are an insulin pump user you will be unable to hide your diabetes, because there will be questions about why you have this machine attached to you. A white adhesive cannula stuck on your body is going to be a dead giveaway, even if you stashed the pump when you popped into the loo five minutes ago. Before you even think about it, removing the cannula is not a great idea for concealing your diabetes, because you will lose some insulin. Also, you will still be left with a section of your skin with the adhesive marks on it, and in all likelihood, a small raised area where the cannula was inserted, called a pump bump. If your partner is not aware of your diabetes, it could be difficult in an intimate situation when your blood glucose levels drop and you need to stop to take dextrose. Be safe and be honest. If your boyfriend or girlfriend is worthwhile, then your diabetes is not likely to be a problem.

My wife knew about my diabetes before we went on our first date and it came as a shock to her when we went to the cinema and I ate loads of her sweets! An even greater shock was when we went to a party about two weeks after we met; I had been working all day and had not had the time for an evening meal. There was nothing to eat at the party and I literally passed out on the floor from hypoglycaemia. No alcohol was involved. In that sense, my wife had a fair warning of what she was letting herself in for, and her threat to me is that, as repayment for all of this, if my retinopathy causes me to go blind, she is going to dye my guide dog pink!

Challenging Diabetes

Most people that I meet with diabetes are living a fairly normal life and challenge their diabetes to fit into their lives. My own view is that this is a good start, but I prefer to positively challenge my diabetes. Some have described my challenges as a mid-life crisis but, in recent years, I have done the Welsh Three Peaks Challenge – walking Snowdon, Cadair Idris, and Pen-Y-Fan in less than 16 hours. I trained for the Three Peaks Challenge, which involves walking the highest peaks in Scotland England and Wales, namely Ben Nevis, Scafell Pike and Snowdon, inside of 24 hours, but this was cancelled because another key team member became sick with appendicitis 48 hours before the event. I have taken up distance running and I ran my first half marathon after just five months of training. All of these things have had a positive effect on my health and my diabetes and it is for this reason that I consider that I positively challenge my diabetes.

My next challenges are to run two half marathons this year, both without having a hypo. I am chair of the organising committee for the Juvenile Diabetes Research Foundation Walk for a Cure in Cardiff, and we aim to double the amount we raised at last year's event. I will, of course, continue working with INPUT diabetes representing them in at the Welsh Assembly, and I am proud to be part of the 2014 JDRF Type 1 Parliament, which is asking politicians and policymakers to help us with funding into a cure for type 1 diabetes. In June 2014, I climbed Kilimanjaro with 18 others who have type 1 diabetes, 17 of us made the summit together making history as the largest team of people with type 1 diabetes to summit together. This trip is important in raising awareness of type 1 diabetes and in demonstrating to everybody that type 1 diabetes is not a barrier to achieving your plans. And now, how are you going to positively challenge your diabetes? Treatment for type 1 diabetes means that you must have replacement insulin. You cannot take tablets and as far as we know, there are no cures at this time. In addition to treatment by insulin, most of us follow a modified diet and my views on this have already been covered in the nutrition section of this book. At the time of this writing the only methods we have for taking insulin are via an injection or the use of an insulin pump. We have seen some developments for inhaled insulin but the uptake was poor, probably for these reasons: Only short acting insulin was available; the inhaler device was huge, and a small suitcase was required to carry the device; and the safety of inhaled insulin in the long term remains questionable. Insulin promotes growth and inhaling a product which promotes growth into your lungs may have adverse side effects in the long term. Before anybody gets too excited by the prospect of inhaled insulin I believe it has now been withdrawn from the market, but keep watching this space since generation one of any emerging technology always has problems.

My journey with diabetes began with a single injection each day. My syringe was a huge glass contraption that was stored in surgical spirit between each injection and the needle was reused many times. I even had a wire brush to insert down the centre of the needle to clean it and clear blockages. We now understand that this system is not appropriate due to increased chances of infection and the blunt-force trauma of reusing a needle causes considerable damage to the tissue resulting in reduced insulin absorption. I should mention that it is painful to use a needle that is as thick as a knitting needle and equally as blunt! Technology has moved on considerably in the last 40 years and today injections are given with a disposable syringe or commonly with an insulin pen.

CHAPTER TEN

DIABETES CARE PLANS

The most common insulin therapy for type 1 diabetes is a basal-bolus regime. This means that you take a short or even rapid-acting insulin to cover meals and high blood glucose levels. This is the bolus part and you also take a long-acting insulin to provide background insulin, which is the basal part. You can associate this with the basal metabolic rate, which is responsible for all of those background activities that your body performs without even thinking about it, such as breathing and digesting food. I used this type of insulin therapy for about 22 years and it works. I was having some considerable challenges with dawn phenomenon and would wake each morning with an elevated blood glucose measurement. I could resolve this by increasing my basal (background) insulin, but in doing this I was experiencing a lot of hypos throughout the day as my background insulin levels were too high after the effects of cortisol and catecholamines had worn off in the mid-morning. One solution for me was to set the alarm and inject a few units of rapid-acting insulin at 03:00 in the morning, and although this worked well, it is not sustainable or sociable.

After 29 years of injecting I went onto an insulin pump, which technically is called Continuous Subcutaneous Insulin Infusion (CSII). This means that I only have rapid-acting insulin and the pump is programmed by me to deliver a constant feed of rapidly acting insulin at varying rates throughout the day and night, acting as my basal insulin. Unfortunately, the pump requires manual programming and you must work out how much basal insulin you need and when you need it. This is the biggest challenge in using an insulin pump, but in my opinion, it is worth investing the time and effort to do this. The value of an insulin pump comes from these benefits: The increased flexibility, the ability to manage my overnight insulin loading to deal with my own diabetes physiology and my improved diabetes management.

There are no positives in life without negatives, and the negative side of the pump is that I need to monitor my blood glucose levels much more carefully now. On a basal-bolus insulin injection regime I could get away with missing the occasional injection because the basal insulin would carry me through and if I did not do a blood test from one day to the next that too was kind of OK. The pump gives me no long-acting insulin and if insulin delivery fails, I am exposed to rapidly climbing blood glucose levels and, perhaps, even DKA in just a few hours. In my experience the most common cause of this is a kinked cannula under the skin surface, which you cannot see, but it slows or prevents insulin delivery. This type of fault typically only occurs when you insert a new cannula (or set) and for this reason, I leave the old set in place until I am convinced the new set is competent. I also try to avoid changing my set at night, preferring instead to time my set changes so that I can observe my blood glucose levels closely in the next four to six hours. On a couple of occasions, I have managed to dislodge a cannula in my sleep, which has lead to a loss of insulin supply and caused rapidly rising insulin levels. On one occasion my pump motor failed, and the pump had to be replaced because it would not rewind to put a new reservoir of insulin in it. In spite of all of these considerations the pump is an amazing device, and I would never go back to injecting insulin on a basal-bolus programme.

I would not wish diabetes upon anybody and hopefully my children will remain free from diabetes, but, if they are ever diagnosed with type 1 diabetes, I will not allow them to be discharged from the hospital into my care, until they have an insulin pump; unless, of course, something better comes along to replace it! I say this to demonstrate to you how strongly I believe that insulin pumps are the most appropriate treatment for people who are proactive in managing their diabetes. This is probably not an appropriate treatment choice if you or your loved one is diagnosed with type 1 diabetes, and you have no experience of living with diabetes. I am well versed in insulin pumps and can revert back to injecting insulin instantly when the pump fails. I would not advocate going onto an insulin pump unless you are confident enough to make the transition back to injections in an emergency. However, if you are living with diabetes and you don't have an insulin pump in your life, please start investigating the possibility. Without my insulin pump and continuous glucose monitor, it would make it very difficult for me to go walking in the hills, to run half marathons, and to climb Kilimanjaro.

Diabetes Cures

As soon as you start searching on the Internet about diabetes, you will be bombarded with advertisements for diabetes cures. Most of these are aimed at people with pre-diabetes or even type 2 diabetes, and I believe that in some cases these can work. However, if you have type 1 diabetes these cures do not address the root causes of the disorder, which is an underlying autoimmune response that has damaged the insulin-producing cells. If we could retrain the immune system to stop attacking the islets of Langerhans Beta cells, there might be some possibility of preserving or even increasing insulin production.

There has been some modest research performed that has demonstrated in postmortem that even people with very long-standing type 1 diabetes retained some insulin-producing islets of Langerhans cells. This is good news because it means that islet cell death may not be complete and absolute. If researchers can find a way of promoting a controlled expansion of population numbers of these remaining competent cells, we might just have a cure. Before you crack open the champagne, consider this: When I was diagnosed back in 1977 everybody told me that we were on the verge of a cure for diabetes, and that it would surely happen in the next ten years. Almost forty years later people are saying that we are having exciting research developments and we could have a cure in the next ten years! I am afraid my hopes of a cure have dwindled since then; nonetheless, I would love for a cure to be found.

I have come to the realisation that the best hope we have right now is probably of having a mechanical cure first. There is a huge effort underway to develop an insulin pump system which can automatically detect glucose levels (technology we already have) and deliver insulin via a pump automatically (also, technology we possess) in response to those blood glucose levels (this is the tricky bit). In addition to this, the insulin pump would also need to deliver the hormone glucagon (the insulin antagonist) automatically to maintain a stable yet dynamic equilibrium blood glucose level. The technical term for this state is homeostasis. Is this likely to happen? The research is progressing well and there have been some early home studies using this system overnight, outside of a clinical setting, which is very encouraging. If the technology can be made smaller and it demonstrates improvement to the patient's health and safety, then I believe it will become the new gold standard in the future.

We should always remain optimistic about diabetes research as the knowledge continues to grow, and you really never know what is around the next corner. After all, the discovery of penicillin in Alexander Flemming's laboratory was the result of a mistake! This teaches us an important lesson for managing our diabetes: We learn more from the mistakes that we make than we do from the successes that we achieve.

Alternatives

There is no alternative to insulin replacement therapy. The inability to produce insulin is not consistent with life! The possibility of islets cell transplants remains open which means that we may no longer need to inject but for most people the cost benefit analysis does not work in their favour because typically after transplantation you need to take life long immune-suppressant therapy.

We are seeing some exciting and novel approaches to treating diabetes being developed and trials of alpha-1-antitrypsin as a treatment for type 1 diabetes are offering promise right now but they are still in the trial phases.

Your Treatment Plan

Your treatment plan will be as individual as you are. Your body metabolises sugars, fats and proteins at a different rate than mine. You might have more or less insulin-producing cells still actively working than I have. You might have other conditions that affect your diabetes. I know that theoretically, women typically become more insulin resistant in the luteal phase of their menstrual cycle, which is typically days 14 through 28. Your healthcare team is a great starting place for assisting you in developing a treatment plan, but always remember it is your body and your treatment plan.

Since I have been using an insulin pump I have seen the uptake of insulin pumps gradually increasing. For the hospital that treats me I was the fourth patient to start insulin pump therapy; now they have so many people on insulin pumps that they run special pump clinics. I believe that, ultimately, the majority of people with type 1 diabetes will end up getting insulin pumps. This will be especially true when the closed loop insulin pump and the mechanical artificial pancreas become clinically available. When this happens, the argument about patient safety and reduced clinical costs will help to encourage health insurers and national health care providers like the NHS that this is the most cost effective treatment in the short, medium and long term. At the same time, we will see a decline in DKA episodes, hypos, and of course, long-term complications.

TIP

Insulin replacement is the only way that you are going to stay alive, unless you have an islet cell transplant which requires lifelong adherence to immune-suppressant therapy, or you are participating in a ground breaking study for example – for example there is some exciting research underway using an anti-inflammatory substance called alpha-1-antitrypsin which is showing promising results right now. However until we get a cure or a transplant insulin is the treatment of choice for us all.

It is unfortunately common for people with type 1 diabetes to have eating disorders and a separate presentation of anorexia, called diabulimia, exists where people with type 1 diabetes give inadequate insulin levels to maintain a low body weight. They survive on the very edge of Diabetic Ketoacidosis. It sounds like a quick and tempting fix for weight control issues but this will lead to long term health issues including, loss of eye sight, cardio vascular disease including heart attacks and strokes, damage to the nerves particularly supplying the feet and hands which can lead to amputations. The immediate danger is that with only a small miscalculation those who use this as a strategy will quickly slip into DKA a life threatening medical emergency. You will recall that at the time of my own diagnosis I was in a coma induced by DKA and was given only a 40% chance of surviving.

Ultimately, you need to develop the knowledge, skills and expertise to modify your treatment plan. This means that, instead of phoning your care team to ask how you deal with your situation, you should think about the possible solutions before you phone and then ask their opinion of your proposals when you talk to them. Sometimes, your solutions will be right; other times, they will be wrong, but in trying to formulate a solution before you phone in, you are choosing to take an active role in understanding and managing your diabetes. Ultimately, you will reach the position where the majority of your treatment decisions are based upon your own experiences and knowledge, and you will need less and less support from your healthcare team. When you reach this position, always remember to be humble and ask for help when you need it. There is no shame in asking for help, and the only stupid questions are those that you don't ask!

Diabetes is a complex condition, and we all have much to learn about it. The best way that we can learn is to talk to others living with diabetes, because they will have had similar experiences, and they will have developed strategies to deal with them. We know from clinical evidence that patients who attend clinic regularly have better management of their diabetes. It is thought that this is because these patients are held accountable for their diabetes. I believe that health systems across the world are doing a remarkable job in helping us to manage diabetes, but, as a group of patients, we are very insulated from each other. I think we would all benefit from regular sessions where we could talk about diabetes and be accountable to our peers who are living with diabetes, and these support groups are sadly lacking. An expert patient group of peers, who can talk freely and without judgement about the challenges of diabetes and how they deal with them, would be a powerful tool. Many people have preached to me over the years about their perception of how I should manage my diabetes but very few of them have actually lived with diabetes. When I talk to people with diabetes, I find that there is rarely if ever any judgement, just a mutual understanding and support.

One of my goals is to set up online discussion groups for people with type 1 diabetes to actually talk and listen in small peer groups about diabetes with others who live with diabetes. I realise that Facebook already allows something like this, and it is great, but, in my opinion, the meaning and intention of a person's comments can be difficult to convey in short text messages. I am proposing to arrange people into small groups, so that they can actually talk over an Internet connection on a regular basis to learn from each other and be inspired about type 1 diabetes. They can share strategies and successes because we don't have to live alone with type 1 diabetes. Perhaps, by holding each other accountable, we can all improve our lives living with diabetes.

CHAPTER ELEVEN

KILIMANJARO – DEFYING THE ODDS – SETTING NEW STANDARDS

When I was diagnosed, and through my childhood, diabetes defined many of the things that I could and could not do. Back in the late 1970's and early 1980's insulin and food regimes were very rigid and participating in sport often led to hypos and from an early age I watched others participating in sports from the sideline. Many people told me that I would not be able to do adventurous things because of the risk that I would have a low blood glucose level whilst participating and that would be a risk to my life. By the time I was in my late teens I had reached a rebellious phase and I started to participate in a variety of unusual sports. This included disappearing into the hills for a few days with the worlds largest ruck sack, wild camping as we trekked through the countryside, kayaking and even for a brief period, rock climbing, I even became an instructor teaching children the fundamental skills of bouldering and abseiling.

It is only on reflection that I now understand that all of these sports were in some way pushing the boundaries and limitations that others had placed upon me, it was a way of demonstrating that diabetes is not a barrier unless you allow it to be. However, as time went by I started to train in Karate and I spent 3-4 years where I would train 5 times a week and the outdoor pursuits slowly stopped. It was not that I was no longer interested; it was simply that I did not have the time, although it was always there in the back of my mind that I wanted to return to my outdoor pursuits.

I watched from the sidelines as a friend completed the 3 Peaks challenge and I was reminded of those early times when I could not participate due to my diabetes. I began to think that the 3 peaks challenge would be a great test of how far I could push the boundaries of my diabetes and we put a team together, deciding that we would do the 3 peaks challenge. At about this time my brother, Mark and his partner Linda, had decided to climb Kilimanjaro on an expedition hosted by a mutual friend, Eric Edmeades. I was invited to go too but I had developed retinopathy and all of my investigations suggested that this would prevent me from safely reaching the summit. Therefore I declined the offer and continued to train for the 3 peaks. After just 8 weeks of training we set out on a trial run, to complete the Welsh 3 peaks – which means we climbed the highest peaks in North, Mid and South Wales in less than 16 hours – this includes the time to travel between these peaks.

We had a late start to the day, we had not trained nearly enough and some of the equipment we had was not adequate for this event and perhaps most importantly in addition to all of the walking, we were taking it in turns to drive between the peaks. Needless to say we did not achieve our goal and we had a lucky escape as the weather changed on the second mountain (Cadair Idris) and mountain exhaustion began to set in for me. I had already experienced a large number of hypos during this event by this time and I was battling to keep my blood glucose levels up, the supplies of glycogen in my liver and muscles were already exhausted and as the temperature dropped my core body temperature began to fall with it. Simply put it was time to get off of the mountain and quickly before we had a medical emergency on our hands.

We did not achieve our goal that day and we went home feeling dejected and upset, however I had learned lots of valuable lessons and I decided to start asking better questions about how I could achieve this endurance challenge. It was then that I enlisted the help of the amazing medical experts at Runsweet, and Dr Alistair Lumb gave me some crucial and valuable advice about how to manage my diabetes during this type of endurance event. I also replaced some of my equipment and decided that in future I was no longer going to carry a flask, instead I would carry a stove so that a hot drink could always be made available. I also decided that GPS was not worth having and that I needed to brush up on my map and compass skills.

We continued our training and 4 months later we repeated the challenge, this time we were ready and we completed the event in 15 hours and that even included a stop for a meal. The lessons we were taught by our previous experiences had prepared us well, and reinforced my own philosophy that mistakes are valuable lessons. We continued to train and prepare for the 3 peaks challenge and in June 2012 we were ready to go. Suddenly 48 hours before the event one of the team member's, Dennis, developed appendicitis and was rushed into hospital. The event was cancelled as we had trained together and we were not going to do this without a vital member of our team.

It was only a couple of months later that I had yet another invite to climb Kilimanjaro, the universe was clearly telling me that this was something I should be considering. I consulted with my medical team and my Ophthalmic surgeon confirmed that spending time at an altitude of 5895 metres would put my vision at serious risk and there is no way that I should participate in such an event. I had already been reading the research material on this very subject and I felt that his advice was well considered and so once again I turned down the opportunity. In my heart I really wanted to climb Kilimanjaro having heard my brother speaking of his time on the mountain was contributing to my desire to participate in this incredible challenge. Once again the memories of my childhood were coming to the surface, all of those times in my childhood when I could not participate in sports and events and I was feeling that in spite of all of the advances in diabetes management and technology, nothing much had really changed.

As Dennis recovered from his appendicitis he persuaded me against my better judgement to take up running. You need to understand that I am not a runner, I have never been a runner and I never wanted to be a runner. Yet one evening after too many glasses of wine I agreed to train for and run a 5 Kilometre race (3.1 miles). I think that even now Dennis is more shocked that I agreed to do this than I am. To my surprise I found I actually enjoyed running and within just 6 months I was running my first half marathon. My goals for running my first half marathon were simply to cross the finish line and to do it without having a hypo. I was successful on both counts and I had raised some money for JDRF whilst doing this.

About the same time I was also chairing the organizing committee for the JDRF Walk for a Cure in Cardiff. The event had not be run for a number of years and just 3 weeks after the half marathon we hosted a successful walk, once again raising funds for JDRF. Following the success of the walk I received a call from Adele from the events team at JDRF. She told me that in June 2014 a world record breaking attempt to get the most people with type 1 diabetes to the summit of Kilimanjaro was going to be happening and she asked me if I would be interested in joining. My initial reaction was I would love to... ...but I am afraid that my diabetes complications will prevent me from joining you, I found myself saying, "that sounds amazing, can you reserve me a space please, I have some complications of long term diabetes that might prevent me from going but I will seeks medical advice and confirm my place with you within two weeks".

There were several things that were different about this trip from the previous invites I had to climb Kilimanjaro, there would be twenty people with type 1 diabetes together, there would also be a diabetes consultant, a diabetes specialist nurse (CDE), a dietitian and 2 GP's with us on the mountain. If I was ever going to climb Kilimanjaro, this was the right time. I phoned my own diabetes consultant to discuss my upcoming climb and he immediately told me that he could see no reason why I should not go but this was outside of his expertise, he did tell me to speak with the ophthalmic surgeon who had already operated on my eyes a number of times to preserve my vision, before I confirmed my place.

The ophthalmic surgeon once again told me that this trip might mean that I would never see again. If the already damaged blood vessels in my eyes were further compromised by the effects of altitude I could get a severe bleed into my eyes, if this occurred over a part of the eye called the macula then the loss of vision could be permanent. The surgeon went on to explain that because my macula is already affected by diabetic retinopathy that we should not discount this as a risk and that climbing at this altitude should be avoided. I had spent a number of years looking into this exact question and had seen a lot of research theories but never any evidence that suggested the number of cases that this happened in. To put it another way I knew the theories but I could not work out the likelihood that those theories might actually become the reality for me. My next question I asked was how many people with diabetic retinopathy and/or macula oedema had actually suffered from hemorrhages in the eye leading to sight loss by being at altitude? His answer gave me the hope I was looking for, he told me that there was no data to support the theory because not enough people with diabetes and retinopathy/macula oedema have climbed at altitude.

Suddenly I understood the advice I was given not to climb Kilimanjaro was good conservative advice but based purely on a hypothesis. I have been around medical and engineering data for most of my life and now I understood that this really meant I was given advice to keep me safe and to keep my medical team safe. Strictly speaking the textbook says I should never climb to or spend time at altitude, but the reality is that we must each balance our own attitude to risk. I was not yet ready to confirm my place on the trip, I needed more clarification of the risk to my eyesight and I wanted to understand how I could best manage my diabetes on this challenge.

I already knew of Dr Ian Gallen's work at Runsweet from my 3 peaks training when I learned that he was the chief medical advisor on our trip to Kilimanjaro. I asked my Doctor to refer me to Dr Gallen and my request was refused for bureaucratic reasons. I could demonstrate that I had a distinct clinical need and even my Doctor agreed that this was the case but he told me that because of the way that the financial systems in NHS Wales work I could not be referred to a consultant in NHS England. You will understand by now that instead of arguing with my Dr who was clearly uncomfortable with the situation I found another way to make this work. I phoned Dr Gallen's secretary and she told me of his private practice and ten minutes later I had privately arranged an appointment that I was going to pay for – the cost was going to be in the region of £100. Just one week later I had driven 130 miles and paid my fees and I sat in the best diabetes consultation I have ever had in my life. This consultation was not about my HbA1c, it was not about my cholesterol or my blood pressure it was how all diabetes consultations should be, it was about me and my diabetes, it was about how I manage the challenges of living with type 1. Dr Gallen went on to explain that there were risks associated with being at altitude to everybody and these were elevated in people with type 1, however there was never going to be any guarantee that I would or would not be affected by altitude or that my retinopathy was going to be made to deteriorate. Dr Gallen told me that my risk of suffering any trauma in my eye was minimal because we would be taking a route that allowed plenty of time to acclimatise to the altitude and that we would only be spending a little time at the summit. He could give me no guarantees but based upon the presentation of my diabetes, my management protocols, the relative stability of my eye disease and my fitness levels he felt that Kilimanjaro was not out of the question.

I had reinforced some vital personal philospohies that day, the quality of your life is not just a reflection of the quality of the questions you ask, it is also about finding the right people to ask. Following this consultation I drove back home and we spent a week discussing the implications of climbing Kilimanjaro. Let us not under estimate this challenge – people can and do die climbing Kilimanjaro. This was going to be both an exciting and terrifying challenge, I had never walked at altitude, I had never met the people I was going to climb with and we had no idea how my diabetes was going to behave at altitude. On the positive side this team were going to be amazingly prepared and the mutual and medical support was going to be amazing.

I had only just completed a half marathon and I spent the winter months of 2013 and early 2014 training for my next half marathon, which was scheduled for the first weekend in March. Late in February I joined two others from the Kilimanjaro group in North Wales for a training weekend to walk in Snowdonia National Park, luckily for us Pete has a holiday cottage in the region and he invited us to stay. The weekend went well and I left with a renewed confidence that this trip was going to be outstanding, I had only spent 2 days away but this was the first time in many years I had spent any time in the company of others who also live with type 1 diabetes; the value of this mutual support was amazing and should not be underestimated. Type 1 is an invisible condition and those of us who have it do an amazing job of living with it, but to actually spend time with people who really understand the challenges and experiences that you have is incredible and in my opinion is the best therapy for diabetes. During this weekend training session we had walked a little but more importantly we had talked a lot about our own coping strategies for diabetes; after all there is no other condition where the patient is expected to continuously recalculate and modify the dose and timing of medications that are essential to keeping you alive. Typically we battle through everything that diabetes throws at us in isolation, people that don't have type 1 may share some sympathy with you but spending time with others who live with it is amazing, they share a similar determination, understanding and for once there is no judgment, just an open and friendly exchange of ideas about how to manage diabetes. If you have type 1 Diabetes then one of the very best things that you can do is to spend time with others who also live with it.

Late in March we had another training weekend, this time it was an official event. Seventeen of us travelled to North Wales and together with some of the medical team, and some mountain guides from the trekking company that we would be using, we spent a couple of days walking in the mountains. The talk this weekend was split almost equally into two main topics; climbing Kilimanjaro and living with type 1. The weekend was an incredible success and my only regret was that many members of the team could not join us on this event. I left that training session knowing that I was climbing Kilimanjaro with the right team, we had instantly formed an amazing team spirit; one of the mountain leaders observed that he had rarely, if ever worked, with a team that had such amazing team spirit.

We each continued our training and there were a few more informal meetings of the guys, some of which I could make, some of which I could not. By now I had changed my exercise routine, for the moment at least running was on hold. When I had a few hours to spare I was out walking in the hills, living only a few miles from the Brecon Beacons was a huge advantage. My own experiences of both the 3 peaks challenge and long distance running were teaching me how to modify my insulin and carbohydrate intakes for a huge endurance event like this. For me personally I use an insulin pump and an hour before I walk, and for the duration of any ascent, I reduce my basal insulin to 20% (e.g. an 80% reduction), I do not bolus for any carbohydrates eaten during this time. As I reach the summit I give 1 unit of insulin and I change my basal insulin to 80% of my normal dose (e.g. a 20% reduction), I continue on this reduced basal reduction until 03:00 the following morning to prevent night time hypos. During the descent phase and after I finish walking I give bolus insulin as normal. This method works really well for me and I was able to demonstrate this by using a Dexcom continuous glucose monitor which is a self funded technology that I chose to use.

Late in the preparation for this challenge my brother, Mark, decided that he wanted to come and climb Kilimanjaro with me. By now he had already climbed it on 2 previous occasions although using different routes from the one we were going to climb and I am not sure if he wanted to climb Kilimanjaro again, if he wanted to spend some time with me or if he was climbing with me because he wanted to make sure that I would be OK. Regardless of his motives it was great news that he was coming and that we were going to climb this amazing mountain together. It was just another way to make climbing this mountain even more special.

As the countdown to the climb began we all started to get nervous about the challenge ahead. There were going to be twenty of us with type 1 climbing together and 15 people without diabetes, those we affectionately termed the muggles. With just a few weeks to go one of our team members was having some difficulties with her diabetes management and she suffered a couple of serious episodes of hypoglycemia, low blood glucose levels, requiring help from others whilst on training – this really could happen to any one of us The medical team decided that this was too much of a risk for her and for us, suddenly our team was down to 19 people with diabetes. It was a devastating moment when we were told this news, for her and for us and yet this amazing young lady plans to climb Kilimanjaro next year, proving that even when diabetes changes your plans it really does not stop you.

I had met about half of the team members through my training but the first time that I met some of the team was at Heathrow airport. Other members of the team were going to meet us in Tanzania as they were travelling in from Canada and the US. It was an emotional moment when I said goodbye to my wife and daughters to board the plane. My daughters had heard some horror stories about climbing Kilimanjaro and they were becoming upset and begging me not to go, my wife was her usual amazing self, taking it all in her stride, comforting our children and dealing with her own emotions.

You should know that the things that I achieve in my life are only possible because I have the most amazing and supportive wife and my daughters are truly remarkable. As a family we have always shared the positive and negative aspects of diabetes and we often talk about the things that might happen to me because I have diabetes, and as I said goodbye I explained to them that one day diabetes might mean that I lose my eyesight or my kidneys may be severely damaged and I might need dialysis which would mean that I could not participate in these adventures so easily and that I need to seize the opportunities now. The lesson for us is that we need to make the most of every single moment that we have together and we must make opportunities to do the most amazing things that we can imagine with the time we are given. I truly hope that this lesson travels with them forever so that they can live extraordinary lives, my plan is to lead by example.

Our flight took us to Nairobi and we then caught a connecting flight to Kilimanjaro International Airport. This connecting flight was an amazing experience as we flew past Kilimanjaro and it's sister peak Mwenzi and we could see the summit just a few thousand feet below the aircraft. As I sat looking out of the window I felt both humbled and privileged as I thought that in just 6 days I would stand on that summit looking down at the clouds below my feet.

Upon arrival in Tanzania we travelled to a hotel to rest for the night, sort out our kit and equipment and to receive briefings on how the trip was going to be organised and what we should expect. This was the first time the whole team, of thirty-one, were together. It was also Kris' birthday and we celebrated with nervous anticipation. As the briefing was delivered Henk, our mountain guide, made it clear that this was our chance to talk about the summit, he told us that after this conversation we were not to talk or ask about the summit again until summit night. These briefings included topics as diverse as toilet facilities on the mountain, which varied between barely acceptable and rudimentary, washing facilities that for the most part consisted of a shallow bowl of warm water each morning, assigning us to medical professionals who would help us with our diabetes care. The medical team led by Omar Mustafa gave us a briefing about how our diabetes medical care would be arranged and what we might expect. One moment remains me about this briefing when we were suddenly advised by Vicky, our dietician that we needed to consume a Mars bar every hour whilst walking to prevent hypos; the looks on our faces were incredulous as we calculated that meant we needed about 40 Mars bars each. Between 19 of us with type 1 diabetes we needed to buy 760 Mars bars and the only shop we would have access to would be the small souvenir shop at Marangu gate, I should remind you that Tanzania is a 3rd world country the shops and facilities are distinctly different from any that we have in Western societies. This advice was based upon the research that she had been carrying out about how fuels are burned and consumed on endurance events at altitude and was given in good faith. However, one of the things we demonstrated as the climb progressed was that the evidence and research on this matter did not align with our experiences. We really did not need 8 Mars bars a day each, in fact I never consumed a single Mars bar the whole trek.

The following morning the team signed in to the Kilimanjaro National Park at Marangu gate, our climb would take the Marangu route up the mountain and each night we would be camping in huts on the mountain. Our first day of walking would be in temperatures approaching 40°C and the humidity would be high as we walked through the lush forests that cover the base of the mountain. As we walked we saw small deer like creatures, called Mountain Reed Bushbucks, and Blue Colobus Monkeys were in the trees over our heads. In the UK this would have been an easy walk but we were already at almost 2,000 metres (circa 6,000 feet) and the effects of this altitude, combined with the humidity, heat and the tiredness from the long travelling hours the day before, were making this walk more challenging that I might have expected. On the first day we only walked for about 5 hours before we reached Mandara Huts where we would spend the night.

We learned quickly that there was going to be a standard routine at the end of each day, this would consist of leaving our bags at the hut as we then climbed another 300-500 metres in altitude before coming back to the hut. This was just another way of helping our bodies to adjust to the altitude, we would then get 30 minutes to sort out our equipment and unpack our sleeping bags and to wash. The team would reconvene for the evening meal and a briefing about the following days trek and timings for the day followed this. Finally those of us with type 1 would check in with our medical team where health screening was carried out and our feet were checked. We would discuss the strategies that we had used that day to manage our diabetes and we would also agree the strategies that we would use the next day. The muggles were left to fend for themselves during this time. After this had all happened it would be time for bed and it was astonishing how quickly we became aligned to mountain time, rising with the sun and going to bed as the sun set.

The first night on the mountain was strange, sleeping in a basic hut with 3 other people. I felt almost sorry for Mark who was sharing the hut with us for he was the only one who did not have type 1 diabetes; the rest of us were hooked up to Continuous Glucose Monitors (CGM) and two of us to insulin pumps. After a long day of travel and changes to time zones the previous day, followed by a day of exercise it really was no surprise that between the three of us we had alarms going all night as blood glucose levels rose or fell. In fact James had some difficulty in bringing his blood glucose levels down that night and found it difficult to sleep; of course the elevated blood glucose levels meant that he had to pee a lot too. The next morning Mark complained to me about feeling tired because of all the pump alarms, CGM alarms, toilet trips, hypo treatments and blood glucose testing that went on through the night, my response lacked sympathy as I said to him that he had only one night of these dramas this has been normal for me for 37 years.

We feasted on a carbohydrate-loaded breakfast before we began the trek to Harombo huts. The trek that day would see us break the tree cover and as we gained altitude we would become more exposed to the sunlight. We were warned throughout the whole trek to make sure that we consumed enough water and each day we were given a minimum water ration that we had to consume whilst walking, maintaining great hydration levels is a fantastic way to mitigate the effects of altitude sickness. It was during the second day that some of my fellow teammates began to feel the effects of altitude, causing headaches and feelings of nausea. The guides and porters with us started to demonstrate just how brilliant they were, offering advice, support and encouragement – with constant chatter, calls of pole-pole which means slowly-slowly. As we approached Harombo huts the guides had arrived before us and they could see that we were tired and our spirits were dropping a little, however they remedied this by greeting us into camp with the Kilimanjaro song and a dance that they all performed and encouraged us to join in. In just a few moments the team were back to high spirits and the mood for the night was well and truly set and as we finished celebrating our arrival we stood there with the clouds below our feet watching the sunset and I felt grateful to have made it this far.

We were staying at Horombo huts for 2 nights to allow our bodies to become used to the effects of altitude and this meant that we had an extra half an hour in bed in the morning before we had to trek again. This was seriously time to celebrate! As we began the third day of climbing we knew that we would only be walking for about 5 hours as we were heading to a famous landmark called Zebra rock, named for the black and white stripes that run down this large monolith. The afternoon session was going to be free time on the mountain, time to chill out, relax and even take a cold shower. As we were arriving back into Horombo huts I was walking with Claire and she was devastated as she told me how her insulin pump had failed and she was going to need to revert back to injections. Injections are a much less flexible option when exercising and don't allow us to rapidly change our insulin delivery, so I understand why she was so upset, however I had been using an insulin pump for long enough that my first pump had been replaced as it's warranty had expired some years before and fortunately I had my old pump in my bag as a backup. I told Claire that I had a spare pump on me, at first she did not believe me and when I handed it over she had tears in her eyes, she later explained she thinks that the loss of her pump might have been the end of her trek as her morale had dropped so severely.

The next morning I woke about 30 minutes before the sun came up feeling refreshed and relaxed, ready to face the challenge of the trek to Kibo hut, our final base camp. I sorted my kit out and slipped outside to take some photos of the sunrise. As I came back into the hut I was greeted with some terrible news, Colin had developed an eye infection and although the medical team were giving treatment they simply could not deal with the sudden complexity that Colin had gone blind in one eye overnight. It was decided that he would be medically evacuated down the mountain to a local hospital for immediate treatment. This was a terrible blow to the whole team, Colin is a remarkable guy and truly inspirational in the way he has dealt with the challenges of living with type 1 diabetes, but more than that if there was one person in the whole team who inspired confidence and was going to be the one who never needed any help it was Colin. After a quiet final breakfast together we gathered to say a tearful goodbye to Colin as he was taken down the mountain by one of the mountain guides.

We later learned that Colin was treated in the local hospital but they were poorly equipped to deal with the complexity of Colin's eye condition and he was repatriated back to the UK. It later transpired that the infection in Colin's eye had caused a rare type of trauma and the Doctors in the UK had only ever seen one previous case. The good news however is that Colin received great treatment and his sight is gradually returning to normal and he will be going back to Kilimanjaro next year to finish the job.

By now the landscape was really changing, we were walking through a lunar like landscape, there were few if any plants and the wildlife now consisted of a few birds and some rats that would scamper around if we stopped to eat. We walked through the morning in shorts and t-shirts with the sun blistering down upon us, taking care to make sure we had sun lotion on, sun hats and sun glasses. When we stopped for a lunch break I was stunned as the porters served us fresh hot KFC, yes Kilimanjaro Fried Chicken really was on the menu! I have no idea where that fresh chicken came from how they cooked it in the middle of nowhere at 4,300 metres or how they kept it hot. We were just finishing our lunch when the weather started to change and within a few moments the sun had disappeared and it was snowing. The walk through the wind and snow that afternoon was made so much harder as the path to Kibo Hut, the final base camp, is quite steep and although you can see Kibo hut for hours before you arrive it never gets any closer. The effects of altitude were adding to the challenges that we were facing and as we passed 4,500 metres in altitude it was like somebody had flipped a switch for me. Until this point I had been massively sensitive to insulin, needing only 20% of my basal (background or long acting) insulin and suddenly in the space of a single afternoon I became massively insulin resistant. It was anticipated that this might happen, but it was still a shock as in the space of one afternoon my insulin requirements increased from 20% of basal insulin to a massive 300% of normal basal insulin – that means I need 15 times more insulin. The craziest part of this was that even on this new super dose of insulin my blood glucose levels were still massively high and we began to watch out for signs of diabetic ketoacidosis. Climbing a mountain with high blood glucose levels is challenging enough but the effects of altitude and the medication (Diamox) that I was taking to mitigate the effects of altitude sickness have almost exactly the same symptoms as diabetic ketoacidosis.

As we arrived at the final base camp that night I was feeling exhausted, as my blood glucose levels were massively high and we were all suffering from the effects of low oxygen saturation. Omar had brought a device called a pO2 meter with him, it is used in hospitals to monitor how well patients are oxygenating their bodies. He had been using it to understand how altitude was affecting him and when he tested it that afternoon he was at 86% oxygen saturation, he went on to tell me that if he had a patient in hospital at this level he would put them onto oxygen therapy. I think that the low oxygen saturation and dehydration that is associated with altitude were the drivers behind my massive insulin resistance. In my own particular case my insulin resistance at altitude was following the text book, some others in the team were experiencing similar effects too but at least half of the team were not affected in this way; showing once again that diabetes is a very personal experience.

Our arrival at Kibo hut placed us at the foot of the summit trail, we were now at an altitude of 4750 metres and once again the porters welcomed us with the Kilimanjaro song. It had been a hard day of climbing, we were all exhausted, yet somehow the amazing team of porters and guides were jumping around, dancing and singing and encouraging us to do exactly the same. The guides seemed to know exactly when the team needed a boost in morale and they knew exactly how to do that. Once again we left our kit at the hut and climbed another 300 metres in altitude before we came back to the hut for the evening.

The facilities at Kibo hut are limited, it is a large stone hut with a log burning stove. However because we left the tree line 2 days ago there is no wood or fuel to burn and at this altitude the temperatures are low, it had been snowing all afternoon and it actually felt colder inside the hut than outside. During our afternoon climb we had passed the last water point, this means that it was now so cold that water froze and there were no longer any fresh water sources available, from this point forward the only water you have is the water that is carried with you. Our porters had brought masses of water with them and I can only assume they were find streams as water sources, we had become well accustomed to purifying our water before we drank it. In the absence of any water the toilet facilities at Kibo hut consist of a long drop, this is not a pleasant experience especially when you consider that for some people altitude sickness causes diarrhea and by now all of us were suffering with at least some of the effects of altitude.

We gathered for our evening meal together and the mood was amazing, many of us were suffering with nausea and headaches but that did not stop the team for engaging in lively discussion. Henk advised us of the procedures for the next day, we would do a short acclimitisation hike in the morning arriving back at Kibo hut at midday. After lunch we would have the whole afternoon to rest, we would then have an evening meal and we would head off to bed for a few hours. At 22:30 we would be woken up and we would have 30 minutes to grab a hot drink and a snack and then we would begin our final climb to the summit at 23:00. Henk advised us to go outside and make our peace with Kilimanjaro, he told us that the group were in amazing shape and that we had done everything that was asked of us with a smile, now the difference between making the summit and not making the summit depended on the conditions on the mountain.

At this point I was battling high blood glucose levels and feeling the effects of altitude. The meals on the mountain had been amazing but my diet had changed into a high fat, high carbohydrate diet and at this point I was struggling to consume the food. This was probably a combination of factors; I was feeling nausea from altitude, nausea from the high blood glucose levels and I really could not face any more meals of maize and cassava. The meals on the lower slopes had been great but as we neared the summit the quality and variety of food had diminished; I am grateful for the excellent service that we received and the cooks did an amazing job especially when you consider that they were making almost

300 meals a day and all of the food was carried from the bottom of the mountain.

I struggled to sleep that night, a mixture of anticipation and high blood glucose levels. I needed to pee in the night and I climbed out of my down filled sleeping bag to the awful shock of the ultra cold night time temperatures inside Kibo hut and I walked to the toilet block, as I glanced up at the summit I could see the torches of the guys that were summiting that night. I used this opportunity to give yet another bolus of insulin to try and bring my blood sugar levels down as I thought about the next day and the upcoming summit night. I climbed back into my sleeping bag and spent the next 30 minutes trying to warm back up again.

I woke the next morning to the delights of a high blood glucose level and the feelings of tiredness and exhaustion that go with it. I was greeted with the normal breakfast of porridge and cassava and I struggled to eat any of it as I sat there drinking a mint tea. Within a few minutes we were getting ready for our morning acclimatization hike and we set out practicing our summit walking, the idea was to walk really slowly in single file; ideally our toes should almost touch the heel of the person in front, if for any reason we needed to stop we were to step out of line and join back in nearer to the back. Some of the guides would be at the back of the line to make sure that everybody stayed together.

By lunch time we were back at Kibo hut and my blood glucose levels were remaining really high, I was now giving correction boluses (doses of rapid acting insulin) every hour in an attempt to drop my blood glucose levels. I managed to eat a small lunch that was packed with carbohydrate and I gave

3 times my normal insulin requirements for this. Normally I would not have eaten with my blood glucose levels being so high the medical team were concerned that we needed enough carbohydrates on board to deal with the challenge ahead. At this altitude the body is thought to be unable to burn fats as a fuel source and I knew it was vital to make sure that I had enough fuel to reach the summit. By the middle of the afternoon my blood glucose levels had reached the low 28mmols/l (442 mg/dl) and I was working really hard to bring them down. I was consulting the medical team and we were monitoring for ketones. As the evening meal approached I had been giving insulin shots every hour, on the hour, in case the pump was not working effectively and I was still on 300% of my normal basals; I made a decision that there was no point eating the evening meal, my blood glucose was so high that I would just pee the excess glucose out, losing precious salts and minerals at the same time. I discussed my plan with the medical team and they agreed that this seemed like a sensible suggestion. I joined the team at the last meal and sat there drinking hot water. The last meal before the summit was an unusually quiet affair as each of us worked through our emotional and mental preparations for the challenge that we were going to face together that night.

After a couple of hours of much needed sleep I was woken up for the summit preparation, at this point Chris was putting on his very special summit pants, a pair of pink pants (briefs) that said Ski Bum on the back. The deal was that he was going to pull his trousers down and do a moonie at the summit wearing these pants in some crazy arrangement he had made with friends back home. This whole adventure had been Chris's idea in the first place as part of his 7 challenges on 7 continents campaign and Chris was no stranger to adventure as a person with type 1 diabetes and a professional snowboarder. His crazy pink pants certainly made the 20 guys in our dorm smile.

As we met up for a final hot drink and biscuits my brother, Mark, was struck with altitude sickness and rushed off to vomit. I alerted the medical team immediately and they gave him some medicine to settle his stomach, the decision was made that he should walk at the front, leading the group – limiting the pace to his capability at that moment I had already decided that we were going to summit this mountain together. At exactly 11:00 we began our trek, we each carried 4 litres (almost 8 pints) of water. For me this meant 2 litres in a water bladder, 1 litre neoprene coated water bottle and 1 litre of hot water in another neoprene sleeved bottle. Just 30 minutes into our trek the water bladder had frozen as the temperature dropped to a staggering -20°C, as I checked with other members of the team they were experiencing the same. No amount of insulation or blowing the water back into the pipe had any effect – water bladders clearly are not the way to cope on summit night. The routine for the whole night was that we would walk for one hour and then we would rest for 5 minutes, this was a punishing task and as we became more tired, colder and the effects of altitude had greater effect, we wanted to rest for longer but stopping and resting means that you get even colder and the risk of hypothermia increases.

All of us with type 1 were now focusing on keeping our blood glucose meters close to hand and warm enough that they would actually operate, keeping our insulin warm and for those of us on insulin pumps this also meant keeping the pump and its batteries warm. We achieved these things by keeping pumps next to our skin, the logic here was that our bodies are at 37°C and if our core temperature drops more than 1-2 degrees we will have hypothermia and that is an entirely different medical emergency and we accepted that although the ideal temperature of insulin is considerably cooler than this, in the short term it was unlikely to do any real damage. Another challenge we faced that night was in performing blood glucose tests – taking gloves off to perform blood glucose testing when the temperature is -20°C is less than ideal and exposing the hands to low temperatures can in fact lead to hypothermia. My Continuous Glucose Meter had performed amazingly well throughout the challenge and I elected to trust the data from the CGM on summit night, however I still carried and protected my blood glucose meter as a back up.

After a couple of hours of painfully slow walking we reached Hans Meyer's Cave, this is a major landmark on the summit route and we were given a drink of hot, sweet tea. It was now about two thirty in the morning and we were all feeling tired and it was cold. We knew that the next 3-4 hours were going to be the toughest as the temperature drops in those pre-dawn hours, many of the team were really experiencing the effects of altitude sickness which can include any combination of diarrhea, vomiting, shortness of breath, hallucinations, elevated heart rate and for some of us with Type 1 massive insulin resistance. At this point it was 15 hours since I had last eaten and my blood glucose levels had actually stabilized in target range with the combination of huge doses of insulin, starvation and exercise. I was all too aware that this was working for me but I knew that I was performing endurance exercise in extreme conditions and that the human physiology does not utilize body fat as an energy source very efficiently at altitude (with low oxygen saturation levels).

About an hour after leaving Hans Meyers Cave my hands started to get cold, I was wearing thermal gloves with buffalo mittens over the top. I knew that cold hands could be the start of hypothermia as warm blood from my bodies core would be taken to my hands to warm them up and the cold blood would then be circulating in my core; this was an early warning sign and I needed to act quickly. I stepped out of line and one of the porters was with me as we pushed hand warmers inside of my gloves, the relief was instant but now I had a psychological problem. During the whole trek you are supporting and encouraging your team mates and they are doing the same for you, however summit night is different the team spirit does not leave you but you can only have support from the person in front of you and the person behind, conversation is limited, speaking requires precious oxygen. I was climbing this mountain with a great team, but I wanted to summit Kilimanjaro with my brother and now he was at the front of the line and I was near the back. I told the guide that I was going to summit with my brother and that we were going to catch him. He advised me that this would be hard on me because I was already fighting for oxygen, we discussed it briefly and he could see that I was determined to reach the summit with Mark and we picked up the pace and walked alongside the group until we reached the front again. I was gasping for air but I was in a strong place mentally and my hands were beginning to warm up, I started to feel that unless the mountain decided to give us some additional challenges that I was going to make the summit.

My change of mental state to one of absolute certainty that I was going to reach the summit pushed me through those last hours and strangely I was surprised to learn that I had just reached Gilman's point, the first summit of Kilimanjaro – the time was 05:10 in the morning and the sun was not yet visible, our goal of reaching Uhuru peak for sunrise was definitely a possibility now. Kilimanjaro is a volcano and to reach the highest point means that you must walk around the edge of the crate rim. Mark and I were still leading the team but I was struggling now, even though I was walking more slowly than I have ever walked I was breathing like I was sprinting and things were not getting any better, with each step I was longing for the next rest point; I knew that with every step forward I was one step closer to both a rest and the summit and those drove me to continue pushing through the absolute exhaustion that I was feeling. Finally we reached Stellar Point, the next summit of Kilimanjaro and as I staggered to the signpost in the darkness altitude sickness struck me like a bolt out of the blue, suddenly I was throwing up. Instantly my porter Joseph was with me pulling my back pack off of me, rubbing my back and shoulders and assessing my health, I knew at this moment that he would decide if I could continue or if I needed to descend and there would be no room to argue or negotiate. I sat there for a moment gathering my thoughts, I was determined that my physiology would not stop me from walking the last 20 minutes to the highest summit. I brought my breathing under control and I stood up, Joseph could clearly see that change in me and he told me that now I had been sick I would feel much better and that the summit was only a few minutes away. Sure enough he was right, Joseph now carried my rucksack and I could see the fingers of pre-dawn light in the distance.

Mark had stopped to wait for me and our roles had reversed, just a few hours ago he was being sick and needing some help and now I was in that position and yet now he seemed comfortable with the environment and altitude. We continued our trek and at 06:24 I reached the summit. I shed a few tears as I watched the sunrise on this winter solstice morning from the highest point in Africa. The views were amazing as the sun bathed the glacier in a golden orange light and we could see the curvature of the earth and in the far distance I could see Mount Kenya beneath us. As more and more of the team joined us people were taking a few moments of quiet gratitude and tears were flowing as we thanked each other for the amazing experience that we had joined in together. We had defined new standards in diabetes, never before had such a large team of people with type 1 diabetes joined together and performed and climbed Kilimanjaro, we had expanded not just our own knowledge of what is possible with type 1 diabetes but we had also educated an entire medical team in the amazing tenacity that you need to beat diabetes every single day. I am certain that it is this amazing determination and tenacity that we use every single day that drove us to the summit.

As I left the summit sign Siobhan, the team Diabetes Specialist Nurse was just reaching the summit. I stood there in awe of her as she had placed the needs of every single one of us before her own needs throughout the whole trip. I also knew that this summit night had been really hard for her, she had battled altitude sickness the whole way and she told me how her guide had nursed her through the night and encouraged her to achieve this amazing goal. As she stood there telling me this with tears flowing down her face she said "I don't know how you guys have done this, living with the challenges of diabetes is always difficult but as I struggled up this mountain last night I kept thinking of how much harder it is for all of you; you are all amazing". I know from our conversations that Siobhan has been a DSN for many years and has an amazing knowledge of diabetes and I know that she will take her experiences of our climb back into her everyday practice to inspire others with diabetes to ask questions about what they can do.

All too quickly I had to leave the summit, I was still struggling with altitude sickness and my body was telling me that it needed help, I needed to get down this mountain. As I began to descend I was sick one again, and as I looked up I realised that once again I was at Stellar point. Unfortunately this time I had no amazing goal to focus my attention, I was also now massively dehydrated, in fact it felt like I had severe Diabetic Ketoacidosis, although my blood glucose levels were at 5.1 and I felt so exhausted that I just wanted to stop and rest. I needed fluid and I needed it quickly but most of my water was still frozen. Joseph could see that I needed to get down from that mountain and quickly, he linked arms with me and we staggered down that mountain path together like a cross between an old married couple and a pair of drunks. I believe that the only difference between my summit and descent was that I had now lost my driving focus and this means that the symptoms that I was feeling were suddenly amplified – I know now that I needed to change my mental state, I needed to focus on the celebrations that were going to happen in the coming hours and days but I was too caught up in that moment. Joseph did an incredible job of keeping me safe that morning and when I needed a drink he would get my water bottle out for me, open the lid and on the higher slopes he would even hold the water bottle for me. A little after 09:30 in the morning I walked, hand in hand with Joseph, into the base camp at Kibo hut.

When I arrived at the hut I learned that one of our team did not make the summit, he had developed early signs of hypothermia and had been brought down from the summit. When we checked in on James, he was still fully dressed, wearing hat and gloves inside his sleeping bag and he was still feeling bitterly cold, telling us that he did not know any way to warm his hands up. It was sad that James was unable to summit with us but the important thing was that he was safe and well.

31 people attempted to summit Kilimanjaro on this trip, 19 of them have type 1 diabetes. 29 People made the summit, including 17 people with type 1, that is far beyond the normally accepted levels of success and it is amazing that the 2 people who did not make the summit were not stopped because they have type 1 diabetes, instead it was other external factors; an eye infection and early signs of hypothermia which stopped them this time.

In summary, this expedition taught me a great deal about my diabetes and how it influences my life. I learned a number of lessons about myself on this climb about how I cope with challenges and adversity but perhaps the single most important lesson for me was that the limiting beliefs of others should never define my life and the things that I am capable.

Once again I find that in some strange way I am grateful for the fact that I have diabetes, I may never have climbed Kilimanjaro if I did not have type 1, I probably would not have done this with such an incredible team. I truly believe that in reaching this summit I may have finally demonstrated to myself, and others, that the only barriers to success are our own limiting beliefs or the limiting beliefs that we allow others to define us with.

So what is next? In honesty I have not yet decided but I will continue with my running and my bucket list now has a second climb of Kilimanjaro on it...

CHAPTER TWELVE

DIABETES IS A FAMILY AFFAIR

This chapter is written by those closest to me, who are also living with the trials and tribulations of my type 1 diabetes on a day-to-day basis, as observers and participants in my treatment. They each have a story to tell of how my diabetes has had an impact on their own health, and most importantly, the way in which type 1 diabetes has had a deep and profound psychological impact upon them. To the best of my knowledge, none of us have ever been offered counselling to come to terms with diabetes, and reading these contributions makes me painfully aware that it is a missing link in the management of diabetes. I would like to thank my mum, my brother, my wife and my daughter for contributing to this unique perspective of type 1 diabetes. Each of them tells an amazing story on its own, but combined together we start to understand the impact diabetes has on the whole family.

Mum's the Word
by Eileen Coker

Looking back on old photos of Paul now I can see something was possibly not right with his health, as he looked pale with sunken eyes, but at the time because you are living with it, you tend not to take too much notice. Shortly before the holiday which changed our lives, I was becoming concerned about Paul's weight, and my resolution on our return was to take more care with his diet. Little did I know that it was going to be taken out of my hands, and, after his diagnosis, I felt awful thinking I had tempted Providence.

We had planned a camping holiday with friends to Loch Lomond in Scotland, and en route we stopped overnight in the Lake District, where the children played in a small stream and were soaked up to their waists. The journey to Scotland continued the next day, which I think was a Friday. During the trip, Paul needed the toilet often and even wet himself; I thought he had an infection due to getting wet the day before. The next day he started to feel unwell and appeared to be showing signs of a sore throat. A visit to a local doctor confirmed he had a sore throat, for which Paul was given antibiotics, and then we bought him an ice cream 'to soothe his throat'. The next day Paul looked dreadful, and we decided to pack up the tent and head for home, thinking this was the best place for him as it was now raining and so damp. Whilst packing the camping stuff away in the rain, we left Paul in the car to keep warm and dry. Then I noticed him drinking a bottle of lemonade as if he were in a desert, still not knowing what was happening

I knew nothing of diabetes, but that was about to change.

As our journey home progressed down the motorway, we stopped for fuel. I took Paul to the toilet and had to hold him because he had become so weak that he could not stand or sit unaided. This is when I noticed all his body fat had gone, and he looked like a living skeleton. I was so scared. After this stop we sped down the motorway with no regard for speed limits, and these days we would have set off hundreds of safety cameras. During the last part of the trip, I held Paul on my lap and his eyes were rolling back in his head, and I think now that was probably the start of the coma. I just needed to hold him whilst I still could. On our arrival home, which I think was about midnight, we phoned the emergency doctor. Fortunately, he was there in no time, and he took one look at Paul, telling us to get him to the hospital and not to stop for anything. We didn't even stop for red traffic lights, and the camping equipment was still on the roof of the car. We were so frightened. When we arrived at the emergency room, the doctors and nurses were at the hospital door, waiting for us to arrive. They took a medical history, blood, and urine samples, and very quickly gave us the diagnosis that Paul had type 1 diabetes, or as they called it back then Juvenile Diabetes Mellitus. Although this meant Paul had an on-going condition, the relief we felt was unbelievable.

At the time, I did not understand what type 1 diabetes meant, and I still cannot remember the correct numbers of Paul's blood glucose levels at that time, but I think they had reached over 160 mmol/l (2880 dg/mL). After making sure he was in safe hands, we left for home at four in the morning, returning to the hospital at around eleven. By now Paul had lost the thin, gaunt look from the previous night, and he was now red and plump, but still in a coma. A few days after Paul recovered from the coma when he was feeling much better, he asked me, 'when will I get better?' What can you say? It was a very difficult moment explaining to a five-year-old that he had to live with this condition, and he had to take injections every day for the rest of his life. The staff were very good to us, and I was able to stay with Paul all the time. They made a game out of the syringes, using them as water pistols. During Paul's stay in hospital (about 11 days), we had meetings with the doctors, and they explained how to cope with the diet, testing, and injections. I remember that we learnt how to do injections by practising our technique on oranges.

The first injection I gave Paul was the hardest one to do, but I had no choice since I needed to do this to keep him alive, and, in the end, you do so many that you don't notice them anymore. During the last few days of his stay, the staff asked us to walk Paul to the local shopping centre at lunchtime, and, on our return, his blood glucose levels dropped, and he became hypo. This was done so that we would get to see our first hypo and learn the methods of treating it whilst still at the hospital. The nurse insisted that Paul must drink a glass of milk with sugar mixed into it. I think she regretted this, because the milk came back up faster than it went down, as he threw up all over the floor and the nurse. I recall that anytime we were near a hospital, and Paul became hypo, they insisted that he drink milk with sugar in it. One of the nurses told us that they do this to all patients with diabetes who are hypo, and nearly all of them throw up. We quickly learnt to use glucose tablets instead.

When Paul came home it was very scary, as we were now responsible for his well-being and his diabetes. There was so much to learn and everything needed to be taken on board. The school was very good; every day I went to see the cook to work out Paul's food for the lunch break. I used to go on all of the school trips, because the school was anxious about coping with Paul's diabetes, and I have to say I had some good days out. At the time Paul was diagnosed, my hair was long, reaching halfway down my back, but, within a few weeks, my hair started to fall out by the handful, as my body and mind were adjusting to our new life with diabetes. I had to have my hair cut short to prevent more of it from falling out, and I have had short hair ever since.

At first, we monitored every single thing, buying specialist diabetic foods so that Paul would not feel left out. These were not only expensive, but eating too much has its problems due to the sorbitol content, which causes diarrhoea. I love to cook, so I decided to work out the carbohydrate contents in the foods that I cooked at home, a much healthier alternative. It also occurred to me that, if Paul was unable to eat the same foods or sweets that other children enjoyed, he may rebel and go on a binge, which would not be a good thing. So, he was allowed normal sweets, but we monitored them closely. I hope Paul feels that we had his best interests at heart. One hot summer day, a neighbour knocked on my door to apologise. The children in our street were playing outside, and, when the ice cream van came, she bought them all an ice cream. When she asked Paul what he would like, he said he couldn't, and she felt terrible, but I was really proud of Paul.

At the age of seven, Paul attended a summer camp organised through the British Diabetic Association. It was the hardest week for me, worrying if he was okay, and I spent a few nights crying. However, Paul came back full of confidence, able to do his own injections, which up until then he had refused to do, and it was probably the best thing that happened to him.

Around this same time, it was necessary for Paul to have a small planned operation on his nose. The day prior to his operation, I was told not to visit him on the day of surgery, but to wait until the day after surgery. On the evening of his operation, I had a very strong feeling that I should go to the hospital, so I did. On arrival walking into the ward, which had four beds either side with older women, who had had similar operations, I found Paul in agony. His bed was in the centre, and he was writhing around, and when he saw me, he said, 'Help me. Mum'. I immediately found a nurse who informed me that they did not know how to deal with diabetes (I have to say this was only an ear, nose, and throat hospital), so she phoned the main hospital, and they told her what to do. Paul had not had insulin or food and should have been on a drip to stabilise his glucose and his electrolytes. There should have been a diabetes specialist doctor from the main hospital with him for the day. Subsequently, the nurse told me they would probably discharge him the next day, because they could not cope with his diabetes, and they did. The consequences of that day were frightening, and I wonder what would have happened had I not gone there that night.

From time to time, Paul would wake in the middle of the night vomiting, and his sugar levels would be extremely high with the loss of all body fat. This would happen over a few hours and sometimes we would end up back in hospital. The hospital personnel were great, because if I needed them, all I did was phone, and they would admit him directly onto the ward. This scenario to me was not a good situation for a young child, backwards and forwards to the hospital and away from home. It must have been frightening, so I decided to cope as much as I could at home, and the hospital was very supportive of my decision. It also occurred to me as we started going abroad for holidays that I might need to deal with a crisis during one of these holidays when access to a hospital would have been more difficult to arrange. It was essential that I learn how to manage Paul's diabetes if we were to continue with a normal life.

It is hard to let go as children grow up and become independent, and we were always more worried about Paul. In addition to all of the normal teenage activities, we worried that he would go to a party and become hypo, and would anyone notice? Would they just think Paul was drunk? Happily, Paul dealt with his diabetes well, and problems were minimal.

My advice to parents and newly diagnosed people with diabetes is to take each day as it comes, because with time you learn to cope with the condition. At first, it seems that you will never understand diabetes, but it does become a normal part of life. You can always get help and assistance at the end of the phone from the diabetes clinics, and they have always been brilliant to us. It is also worth developing a great working relationship with your pharmacist for your prescriptions. Once when Paul was unwell, his dad picked up a prescription from the doctors, and when the chemist saw it, knowing Paul was diabetic, realised the doctor had prescribed an unsuitable medicine.

Paul has achieved so much, this includes camping in caves, kayaking, orienteering, a successful career, marriage, and two beautiful daughters. This year Paul completed the half marathon in Cardiff, showing again that Paul never lets the diabetes beat him, he beats it. Well done, Paul, your dad and I are so proud of you.

Diabetes and My Brother
by Mark Coker

If you were with me in July of 1977, you would have been in central Scotland, camping in a big orange tent on the edge of Loch Lomond. It had been a wet few days, and the tent was damp and the wind blowing. My dad's business partner and his family had joined us, and we looked with some envy at their warm, dry caravan.

Over the course of a day or so, everyone began to get irritated with my brother, Paul, as he seemed to keep urinating uncontrollably, wetting most of his clothes and the bed. Paul was complaining of a sore throat, so my parents took him to the local doctor. The doctor wrongly diagnosed a throat infection and gave him liquid medicine with high sugar content to cover the taste. This was a diagnosis that almost cost my brother his life and created a drama, which not only shaped Paul's life, but created a paradigm shift that was to shape our family forever.

Stressed at the continued deterioration in Paul, and not trusting the doctor in Scotland, my parents decided to pack up the tent and head home to Essex, hundreds of miles away. My father's business partner stood in the rain, barely able to see through his rain-soaked glasses, as he bundled the things we had no time to collect into his caravan.

To this day I have no clue why my parents did not go to a hospital in Glasgow. I figure they had no idea of the seriousness of the condition, and how the next few hours would see Paul go from a sickly child to a child in a coma. As we drove through the night in my father's red Mark 3 Cortina, Paul continued getting worse, we sped our way towards home, reaching about 120 mph on the M1, with my mother becoming almost hysterical at the situation unfolding in the car. Upon eventually reaching home, my mother called the emergency doctor. I recall getting into bed as the doctor arrived at the house; this doctor was horrified at Paul's condition and could not understand the Scottish GP's lack of understanding. He instructed my parents to get Paul to the hospital at Basildon immediately, as he suspected Paul had diabetes and would go into a coma and die by morning.

From here on the stress became a bit of a blur; I seem to recall we had a police escort as my dad's car sped through the streets and jumped every red traffic light en route. We dumped the car outside the hospital and carried Paul into the emergency room of Basildon Hospital. Doctors came running from various parts of the hospital as Paul's body began to shut down, and he slipped into a life-threatening coma that was to last several days. Had it not been for the emergency doctor and the rapid reactions, diagnosis, and response from the doctors at Basildon Hospital that night, Paul would have been dead by morning.

At eight years old, I was not allowed into the room where Paul was being treated. I recall that I refused to go home, and I insisted on sleeping on the floor of the hospital day room, maybe in some kind of naive thinking that Paul would recover overnight, and we could all go back to normal the next morning.

Living with a diabetic is strange, as you get into a pattern of seeing everything as balanced and normal (which can be months and months of regular living), then suddenly... Boom, the boss enters back in the room, and diabetes is back controlling the show. Within a few hours, stability, control, and progress vanish to be replaced with mayhem and uncertainty. This can literally be one morning on which a hypo kicks in and an emergency situation arises. With this, all the old triggers fire off, and all the fears and trauma of that day in 1977 appear in a heartbeat.

These kind of uncertainties changed my approach to many things in life and changed my level of risk tolerance in terms of simply doing something. I recall a time that I had a reasonable job and dumped it one day to go off to the USA to spend the summer in Connecticut, doing a Camp America summer camp. All my friends told me I was mad and short sighted to risk my career for a short-term benefit. Had my risk paradigm not been so distorted by living with diabetes in the house, I may well have listened to the rationale of certainty and commitment rather than just going for it and jumping into the unknown. This opened up my world in a different way and took me on a journey as I broke through my comfort zone. I changed my friends to more adventurous risk-takers, and I took a dim view of rules and constraints, finding it hard to hold down a job for any length of time. The good news is that I learnt not to accept things for what they are. I have learnt not only to manage crisis, but to dance with it in some kind of harmony, almost to the point where I would sabotage things, jobs in particular, because I craved uncertainty. Such is the blueprint ingrained on my mind, and I believe these attitudes came from the trauma of 1977.

In the UK, July and August sees the long summer break from school, a time to enjoy days of childhood innocence. This was not for me in the summer of 1977, as the summer was a battle for my brother's life; the entire focus was around doctors and hospitals. Paul was in a coma for what seemed like an eternity to my young mind, and we had been told he had a 50 to 60 percent chance of never recovering. Thankfully, he did start to recover, and with it the roller coaster of remission and illness began of good days and bad days as the blood sugar levels peaked and troughed like an ocean in a storm. Sunken dark eyes of dehydration, fingers and arms filled with pin pricks from blood tests and countless saline drips and insulin injections reflected Paul's condition.

The nurses in the hospital trained us all to recognise the issues of living with diabetes. I volunteered to learn how to deal with the constant injections, spending hours injecting oranges with syringes filled with water in order to learn the process of injecting. I learnt how to get the air bubbles out, what quantities of insulin were safe, and how to measure it. It may not appear much to some people, but, to an eight-year-old child, it was fairly overwhelming. I felt however that, if Paul had to live with this, I needed to understand it as it may make the difference that could keep him alive.

By the end of the summer of 1977, I returned to school with my life changed forever. I don't recall exactly when Paul returned to school, but I do remember other kids harassing him about his issues with sugar consumption. From here on, I became protective of Paul, always wanting to check on him in break times to see if he had the snacks considered essential to maintain his glucose balance.

Looking back I can see that Paul also had a massive issue with nasal mucous, but we did not make the connection at the time to dairy intolerance. However, he was called the snotty nose kid as this green mucous reached from nose to floor on a regular basis. At school I began getting into trouble for having fights with kids that were bullying Paul. I could go into the theory of why I believe milk-based produce caused the mucous and the link with the onset of childhood diabetes, but there is enough material there for an entire book. In short the doctors of the 1970s decided not to look at diet-related outcomes and instead admitted Paul to hospital for minor surgery.

This minor surgery was a drama in itself. I went to school as usual, thinking Paul was in safe hands, totally unaware Paul was being pinned down by nurses in the hospital and refused his insulin. I was horrified to learn later that Paul had a life-threatening experience at the hands of an uneducated medical staff. All the gratitude I had developed for them vanished, as I faced the reality that even those we trust to understand diabetes within a hospital had to ask my mum to take Paul home, because they did not know what to do with him.

As humans we seek to balance uncertainty with certainty. For many years, I sought certainty by protecting my brother, by defending him from bullies and by looking out for him all the time. Thinking back, I suspect this is also why I began working in the family business. My father was always stressed about money and work, so by working there not only did I escape my fear of having a boss, I could also look out for my dad and help him. My parents had a lot of stress placed on them by Paul's condition, and I felt that maybe by working hard in the business and making a difference that I could help the business to grow before I ventured off on my own journey.

On reflection, many of my choices, decisions, and reactions have come from the event that changed my view of reality in 1977. Arguably, this is a place of fear and lack, fear of losing people close to me, a pain inside that I'm somehow not good enough, because I did not prevent that awful situation or at least do something to prevent the situation escalating to death's door for Paul. Even when it came to personal relationships, I avoided any situation that may make me interdependent on another for many years, possibly for not wanting the risk of suffering a loss that could come with any illness. I learnt being close to people meant pain. Therefore, I did not date or have girlfriends until well into my twenties, before then I was always retreating into my own safe space. The further away from people being in my world I could be, the more I could reduce a repeat of the journey of the past, and the more time I would have open to me if Paul needed help.

Since that time, I have been blessed with being with Linda, who is a leading specialist in early years education. She has helped unpick things and replace issues with positive meaning from the imprint years of my early childhood. These issues have extended to the impact the tremendous stress Paul's situation placed on my parents, and the way it influenced their treatment and interactions with me. This is stuff I would never have picked up on without Linda's incredible insight into how childhood experiences influence adult life and allowed me to find ways to mitigate it. Such processes not only deal with the bad stuff but create a profound sense of gratitude for the way things are.

There is a great deal more awareness of diabetes these days. Back in 1977, we had limited counselling; in fact, some healthcare professionals had no clue about the condition, so what hope did the wider family, friends, and community have. Teachers in school had no idea either, as I even had a teacher approach me in school, saying that my brother was unwell and did I know what to do. This may sound a little odd these days but back then, based on the experience with the doctor in Scotland and given my daily exposure to this condition, I would suggest I had more awareness of what to do than the average doctor, even though I was not yet a teenager.

After leaving school, there was a kind of acceptance whereby I realised I could not control things and had to go off to my job and daily business, simply trusting things would be OK. The issue is that, the day things do go wrong, all the old anchors that paved the past come folding back.

Having a brother with type 1 diabetes is challenging when it comes to social acceptance. I have noticed, time and time again, how others expect of Paul the same as they would anyone else; given that, for the most part, since the condition is invisible, other people do not give him the care and consideration he needs and deserves. On the one hand, I know Paul wants to fit in and not be labelled, but, on the other, I know his condition is arguably a disability equal to missing a limb. Yet, a person with a missing limb would get far more consideration from society in terms of expectation, because that is a very visual condition. The hidden nature of diabetes is perhaps the advantage and, at the same time, the disadvantage of the condition. Type 1 diabetes is very much a disability of considerable consequence. Even in the modern workplace today, I would suggest a majority of employers would not really understand the issues and challenges of their diabetic employees, and I would very much doubt the knowledge of many work-based appointed first-aiders would recognise issues and be able to deal with them.

In Paul's case, I know he can be his own worst enemy sometimes, since he rejects the label of being diabetic and attempts to always fit into behaviour that would normally be expected of a fit and healthy person. One thing I learnt from twice summiting Mount Kilimanjaro is the only way to reach your full human potential is to be open and honest with everyone that enters your team, and always, always ask for help at the first sign there may be an issue. It is amazing how asking for help not only increases your chances of success in any situation, but it actually bonds teams and creates shared values and sense of purpose. If I could give you one piece of advice about living with somebody who has diabetes, it would be this, check in with the person with diabetes every time you can, look them in the eyes, check for tell-tale signs of blood glucose imbalance, and learn to recognise the subtle signs that something is not quite right. Make sure you question things that do not seem quite right and cross check. Someone with a blood glucose imbalance can give you incorrect feedback, so never be shy in cross-examining them to see if you get a coherent response, and that it is consistent. Do not wait an hour, as an hour can be the difference between minor intervention and a medical emergency.

Diabetes and my Husband
by Denise Coker

I first met Paul at the very end of 1990, we were both working part time in a shop whilst still at college. Paul would often walk through my department to get things from the stock cupboard, always smiling and saying 'hi' as he went by. Eventually, he would pop down in his breaks and help me to tidy up. We'd chat as we worked, and he would mention things in his conversations that were a little odd coming from a teenager, such as he was not really into parties, didn't drink alcohol, and was careful with what he ate. I can remember clearly being up on a stepladder one day, chatting with him as we tidied and asking him outright if he was diabetic. He looked surprised that I had guessed his condition, truthfully, so was I, as I knew very little about diabetes, only knowing snippets I'd picked up as part of a health questionnaire training course I'd been on.

As time went by, we spent more and more of our free time together; his diabetes was never really discussed during these times, and I never thought to ask. I do have a very vivid memory of my mother asking me if I cared for him, as I was 17 and quite embarrassed being asked such a forthright question. I answered truthfully that I did, but I didn't think he felt the same. My mum obviously saw things differently, and she then asked me not to invest my heart with him. I asked why, and she replied because of his diabetes. My mother was scared that her daughter would end up alone because the boy she adored would die because of his diabetes! This really scared me, and I started researching diabetes. It was now 1991, and the Internet was not yet in existence. I had to hit the medical texts, which was not an easy task. During my research, the words blindness, amputations, heart attacks, strokes, impotence, and early death kept recurring – truly terrifying information. Nowhere could I find any practical advice, sensibly and calmly given. I knew no other diabetics I could ask and was too shy to ask Paul. Despite all the scares, I decided that if Paul ever wanted to go out with me, I would more than happily agree. In my mind, I had decided that a few years of happiness with him were better than none, and I had accepted 100 percent what the books had to say about diabetes.

On July 11, 1991, Paul and I went out for a walk, as we often did. We walked miles and miles in the hot sunshine, no food and no drink, a recipe for disaster. We sat down by the side of a lake, and Paul rested his head on my lap, which was very unusual. He often showed me signs of emotional affection, but this was the first time it had manifested itself physically. Initially, I was thrilled by the closeness, and the fact that he had apparently dropped the last barrier between us. As time went by, Paul's speech was getting less and less guarded, and he was also getting very tired and, eventually, fell asleep on my lap. I let him sleep for a short while, but I was very nervous. I knew something wasn't right but didn't know what. I tried to shake him awake but was unable to, and finally I got water from the lake and threw it over him, which worked. I managed to pull him upright, and we started the long walk home. During the walk, he kept putting his arm around me and being unusually affectionate; instead of being flattered by this, I was more scared, as it was distinctly out of character. I kept asking him if he was OK, and he would always answer that he was fine. Eventually, as he put it, he asked me out to stop me from nagging! When we finally got home, I gave him a lot of juice to drink, thinking that he was probably dehydrated from the long walk and sun; of course, this made him feel a lot better, but I didn't realise at the time that this was because his sugar levels were rising again. It wasn't until months later that I realised he had been low at the time, and it took a few years until he actually admitted that he didn't remember asking me out!

One of our first dates had been to the cinema, and I turned up with a big bag of sweets, confident that they would mostly be for me, after all Paul was diabetic and wouldn't like the sugar and would leave my sweets alone. Wrong! He happily ate his way through the majority of my sweets with, what seemed at the time, no ill effects. Obviously, he must have dosed for this later. From then on, I always ensured I had sweets for the both of us.

About two weeks into our relationship, we were invited to a friend's birthday party, and Paul drove to my house, leaving his car parked at the end of the drive. The party was nothing unusual, with party snacks and fizzy drinks, and alcohol for those who wanted it. We both snacked a little whilst sitting on the floor chatting. As the evening wore on, Paul got more and more affectionate, pulling me into huge hugs, telling me how much he cared for me and, generally, seeming like he was getting drunk. I knew he hadn't been drinking, but I still didn't know how to recognise a low when it was happening. Very quickly, Paul was incoherent and drifting in and out of consciousness; luckily, the host of the party recognised the symptoms (his gran was a type 2 diabetic), and he tried to force water and sugar into Paul's mouth. This proved to be a very bad idea, as we all got showered in sugar when Paul spat it back out. By this point, all the sugary drinks had gone, and my friend drove the wrong way down a one-way street to get more cola. Whilst he was out his girlfriend called my mum and explained what was happening and also called Paul's parents. We, eventually, got the cola inside Paul, and he gradually returned to normal. Paul's parents arrived at the party, understandably worried. On quick examination, they could see that Paul was doing OK, and drove us back to my house to pick his car up. This was not the ideal way for them to meet their son's girlfriend!

This situation served many purposes, since it made me fully aware that Paul was a man with diabetes, and that, if I wanted to be with him, I had to be with his diabetes too, warts and all. It also made me realise that, I knew nothing about his diabetes and at the same time, it made Paul realise that he would need to educate me. From then on I always had something with me in case he went low, sweets, dextrose, drink, any and all. That party was very pivotal for both of us, as we realised that the diabetes couldn't stay in the shadows. I needed to be introduced to it and accept it, understanding that it meant that the man I was hoping to be with forever may not be able to father children, could become blind, could lose limbs, and could die young. I'm still not sure I accept that 23 years later, but I knew then Paul wasn't his diabetes, as he was much more than that: He was funny, cute, intelligent, and someone I loved who just happened to be diabetic.

I have been with Paul since I was 18, and he was 19 years old, and together we have faced many things, all of which have had some effect on his diabetes or on how we view his diabetes. Whilst still early in our relationship, Paul went away to university. It was too far for me to visit him regularly, and long-distance relationships are challenging on anyone.

He was spending many hours studying and as many spare hours as he could working in a bar. These erratic hours and pressures were added stresses to him, his diabetes, and our relationship. Luckily, we coped with all issues that came our way, and I didn't have any of the usual girlfriend worries – will he find someone new, will he cheat, will he stay there? My worries were bigger – what if he goes dangerously low? Who will look out for him? What if he passes out on the way home from the bar, will they think he's drunk and ignore him? I need not have worried though, Paul took relatively good care of himself and his diabetes and came back to Essex.

Shortly after his return, I left for university, again away from home. When I left he was suffering from a cold, insisting it was nothing and that he felt fine. Within days he was diagnosed with pneumonia and pleurisy, and I wanted to come home, but he would not hear of it. He promised he was going to get the proper treatment, but I later found out that this meant seeing a doctor and struggling on in his own way! His early experience with doctors has made him extremely cautious of them, and he never gets himself in a situation where he has to relinquish control to a GP.

On my graduating from university, Paul and I moved in together. This, of course, required more adjustments, including swapping to a new doctor, finding a new diabetes clinic, and also the more practical issue of ensuring that his insulin was always correctly stored. I discovered very early on that the emergency supply that I had of chocolate and sweets had to be regularly checked and stocked up, as Paul, like anyone else, would occasionally crave something sweet to eat, and the supplies would be raided. He still rode a roller coaster of highs and lows, only really monitoring his control when the hospital appointments approached.

In 2002 something happened that changed both of our lives, our daughter Kyla was born. I know that, throughout the pregnancy, Paul felt a mixture of excitement and guilt, obviously excited over the arrival of our first child, but guilt over the fact that any child of ours had a raised likelihood of being diabetic. The pregnancy was relatively easy as was the labour; unfortunately, complications arose during the actual birth, and, only minutes after Kyla was born, she and I were whisked away by ambulance to a larger hospital with a surgery department. I spent several hours in surgery and during this time Paul held Kyla, which gave him a tremendously strong bond with her that still exists today. When Kyla and I were eventually allowed out of hospital, Paul did as much as he could to take the strain off of me. Kyla was a fussy baby and needed regular small feeds and hugs, and Paul did all that he could to help. Of course, Paul was doing all this on top of a full-time job that required long working hours, and he was still concerned about my health.

I think all this worry, stress, and long hours are what brought on an incident that altered a lot of how he reacts to his diabetes. Kyla was maybe five weeks old, and I had only been out of hospital a fortnight and was still in pain and discomfort when Paul collapsed on the floor. Luckily, he did not pass out completely and was vaguely coherent, so I tested his blood glucose levels and saw that he was very low. I raided the cupboards and gave him what stuff we had, but unfortunately his blood glucose levels continued to drop. Kyla had picked up on all the stress and tension and was screaming, I remember putting her in her pushchair and running to the local shop and buying half a shelf of chocolate bars.

On entering the house, I could see Paul was still lying on the floor, a little more with it than he had been but all giggly. I gave him a giant snickers bar to eat whilst I tried to comfort Kyla. He proceeded to eat the bar, wrapper and all! Luckily, this extra amount of glucose seemed to be enough to start bringing him back to normal, and, strangely, as Paul's glucose levels returned to normal, Kyla became less fretful. Once Paul's glucose levels remained stable, I sat down with him, and we talked about the fact that he needed to look after his diabetes more effectively, as I now had a baby that needed my attention too. I could no longer be relied upon to spot the first signs of his glucose levels dropping. From then on, Paul attended his clinics more faithfully, kept better account of his blood glucose levels, watched his diet, and generally reacquainted himself with his diabetes.

In 2004, our second daughter, Cerys, was born. This time I did not need to spend so long in hospital, and the pressure was not there on Paul. Cerys and her dad have a brilliant relationship, but Kyla maintains a special bind with her dad. Now that Kyla was a toddler, we noticed that she often picked up on his dropping glucose levels long before either Paul or I did, as she'd get fussy whilst cuddling him or would try to feed him sweeties. To this day, we have no clue how she knew that he needed to check his glucose levels and adjust them accordingly.

We try to live our life in a healthy manner; we try to eat well and keep active. Paul's diabetes has made us very aware of the importance of a healthy balanced diet, and, of course, we still have times where we eat sweets, take-aways, and fast food, but on the whole we are very aware of the quality and quantity of the food we eat. The girls are fit, trim, and healthy. We are aware that they run a raised risk of being diabetic, and we keep a wary eye out for signs, but it can be almost like seeing signs that aren't there. Cerys, in particular, shows intermittent symptoms, tiredness, general lethargy, confusion, and tearfulness if she doesn't eat regularly, mostly if she has gone through a period of rapid growth. In my bag, I have dextrose at a minimum, often a drink, and some jelly, which serve equally for Paul or Cerys.

Paul's diabetes is very much a part of our daily lives, with nighttime being no exception. At night Paul crawls into bed attached to two devices: his continuous glucose monitor and his insulin pump, both of which seem to have more a presence in the bedroom than us! Paul has been known to snore, which is not good for either of us, and, additionally, his devices beep and vibrate at the oddest times of the night! Paul is used to these sounds and rarely stirs, but I find they disturb my sleep hugely. We have taken to me having his CGM monitor on my side of the bed, so when it beeps or buzzes, I can check it and see what is happening in order to alert Paul to what is needed. Occasionally, we forget, but I think Paul has gotten used to being prodded awake and asked to check his machines, or to having me lean over him and check. There are definitely more than two of us in the bed at night!

I think living with a spouse with diabetes can be a little like living with Jekyll and Hyde. Most of the time, things go along swimmingly, since his diabetes is mostly under control and anything we do is predictable or easily dealt with. During these times, Paul is a calm, easy-going, loving man. When his sugars are out of the normal range for him, it is like living with the Mr Hyde persona, as he is often curt, rude, argumentative, and obnoxious; luckily, these episodes can be easily treated.

I found this Jekyll and Hyde lifestyle very hard when the girls were young. They didn't understand why their usually loving dad was shouting and cross, as they felt like they had done something wrong. With their growing understanding and maturity, they recognise the symptoms and usually tell their dad to do a blood test and treat the problem. They both carry dextrose with them if out and about with their dad and are fully aware of what to buy him if he needs more things. I must admit I do struggle most when Paul's levels are high, since this is when he can become most obnoxious, and it is very hard not to take these things personally. Equally, I have my obnoxious times, and that is what married life is all about, taking all sorts of lows along with the highs, and not just those relating to sugar levels.

Diabetes and my Dad
by Kyla Coker (aged 11)

Hello, I'm Kyla. I am eleven and my dad has diabetes, and I'm going to tell you how it affects me. My dad's diabetes makes me have to be more mature, because I have to take certain precautions, like not climbing all over my dad because it will pull on his pump or his continuous glucose meter sensor, because it will be very painful for him. I also have to be more responsible, because I have to remember to take dextrose with us when my dad and I go out together in case his blood glucose levels go too low, which is rather difficult because I can barely remember to take my own stuff with me. My dad and I don't go swimming with each other very much, because he will lose a lot of insulin. His blood glucose level usually goes high after we swim, and he does not feel well. When he goes high, he can get angry, or he looks really grey, both of which are not pleasant to be around.

On the other hand, there are some upsides to living with my dad's diabetes because I get to go to all these really awesome diabetes events, and everyone at these events is so nice and friendly. I would not meet these amazing people if my dad did not have diabetes.

CHAPTER THIRTEEN

DIABETES RESOURCES

A list of some useful resources for those affected by diabetes.

T1LIFESTYLE

The website to accompany this book is at www.t1lifestyle.com offering support and links to the resources below. Registration is free and gives you access to a growing catalogue of video blogs about various aspects of diabetes.

BOOKS

Dr Richard K Bernstein, *Dr Bernstein's Diabetes Solution: A Complete Guide to Achieving Normal Blood Glucose Sugars*, 4th Edition (2011), ISBN No. 978-0316182690.

Colin Campbell, *The China Study: The Most Comprehensive Study of Nutrition Ever Conducted and the Startling Implications for Diet, Weight Loss and Long-term Health* (2006), ISBN No. 978-1932100662.

Arthur C. Guyton, MD, and John E Hall, PhD, *Textbook of Medical Physiology* (Guyton Physiology) (2000), ISBN Number 978-0721686776.

Gary Scheiner, *Think Like a Pancreas*, 2nd edition (2011), ISBN No. 978-0738215143.

John Walsh and Ruth Robert, *Pumping Insulin: Everything You Need to Succeed on an Insulin Pump*, 5th Edition (2012), ISBN No. 978-1884804120.

INSPIRATIONAL PEOPLE WITH DIABETES

Diana Maynard, a person with type 1 diabetes, who has lost much of her eyesight due to diabetes, and yet she does incredible challenges, such as climbing Kilimanjaro and going to the Everest Base Camp.
expandyourlimits.wordpress.com

Sir Steven Redgrave, five-times Olympic gold medalist in rowing and insulin pump user.
www.steveredgrave.com

Chris Southwell, professional snowboarder with type 1 diabetes doing '7 Amazing Challenges on 7 Continents' to raise funds and awareness of diabetes for research into a cure.
www.7c7a.co.uk.

Melanie Stephenson, a Welsh sprinter with type 1 diabetes.
www.melaniestephenson.co.uk

RESEARCH

Pub Med (great for getting access to research articles).
www.ncbi.nlm.nih.gov/pubmed

The Cochrane Collaboration (great for getting access to research articles).
www.cochrane.org

SUPPLIERS OF MEDICAL EQUIPMENT

Medtronic – Manufacturers of Insulin Pumps & Diabetes Technologies.
www.medtronic.com

Animas – Manufacturers of Insulin Pumps,
www.animas.com

Accucheck – Manufactories of Insulin Pumps and Diabetes Technologies.
www.accu-chekinsulinpumps.com/ipus/

Dexcom – Manufactures of Dexcom CGMS.
www.dexcom.com

Advanced Therapeutics – UK Distributor of Dexcom CGMS.
www.advancedtherapeuticsuk.com

Frio – Wallets for keeping your insulin cool when travelling and have no access to power.
www.friouk.com

MySugr – Tablet and smart phone application for recording blood glucose levels.
www.mysugr.com

GENERAL DIABETES SUPPORT

Insulin Dependant Diabetes Trust
www.iddt.org

Diabetes UK (formerly the British Diabetic Association)
www.diabetes.org.uk

The American Diabetes Association
www.diabetes.org

Diabetes.co.uk (a great site for information)
www.diabetes.co.uk

Juvenile Diabetes Research Foundation (JDRF)
USA site at www.jdrf.org
UK site at www.jdrf.org.uk

Input Diabetes (patient advocates for access to appropriate medical technology)
www.inputdiabetes.org.uk

Insulin Pumpers Blog Site – Everybody should join this regardless of whether you pump insulin or not! The site does not look very sexy, but the information, discussions, and level of knowledge of the users are incredible!
USA Site, www.insulin-pumpers.org
UK Site, www.insulin-pumpers.org.uk

Type 1 University – Partners with Gary Schiener's book *Think Like a Pancreas*
www.type1university.com

The Joslin Diabetes Centre (a fantastic source of information and research)
www.joslin.org

Diabetes Daily
www.diabetesdaily.com

Diabetes Directory
www.mendosa.com

The Grumpy pumper is a blog site written by an insulin pump user in the UK, it is his personal perspective on diabetes.
grumpypumper.wordpress.com